Praise for

Music *and* Canc

A Prescription for Heali

"Over the past several decades, modern medicine has witnessed incredible and exciting advances in the treatment of cancer. These advances have largely focused on improvements in surgery, chemotherapy, radiation therapy, and other novel treatment strategies with the ultimate goal of extending life with cancer, or when feasible, curing cancer. However, it has become clear that simply performing more radical surgeries or administering more aggressive chemotherapy is not the only solution. Cancer patients must be treated as whole individuals taking into consideration their overall quality of life when considering treatment options. Although quality of life has become a major focus of research in the care of cancer patients, improvements in the quality of life have lagged far behind the more tangible treatment modalities as outlined above.

Music and Cancer is a significant advance in improving the quality of life of cancer patients. By approaching cancer from an artistic (musical) point of view, *Music and Cancer* brings to life the humanistic side of cancer care in a way that is easy to understand and enjoyable to read. From diagnosis, to treatment, to the meaning of life with cancer, this book addresses it all. With chapters on topics such as keeping perspective, to end-of-life considerations, *Music and Cancer* takes on the tough and emotional issues related to cancer and presents them in way that is palatable to the reader. *Music and Cancer* is extremely well written, informative, and insightful.

Dr. Nagarsheth is an expert in the field of gynecologic cancer and an accomplished musician/recording artist, and his unique analogies of music and life with cancer are brilliant. Although written for cancer patients and their loved ones, the concepts in this book are easily applicable to all individuals at any stage of life, regardless of disease status. This book is a must read for helping patients and their loved ones manage life with cancer."

Richard R. Barakat, MD
Vice Chair, Clinical Affairs, Department of Surgery
Memorial Sloan-Kettering Cancer Center

"This book is 'music to my ears.' I am thrilled that Nimesh Nagarsheth has written an inspiring and thought-provoking book on the healing properties of music for patients with cancer and their families. My partners and I had the opportunity to nurture Dr. Nagarsheth's interest in woman's cancers during his residency. I am proud that he is merging his talents as a physician and musician in the service of women with cancer.

Gynecologic oncology is a holistic medical specialty in the sense that we provide comprehensive treatment. One doctor acts as surgeon, chemotherapist, and care provider throughout, regardless of the ultimate outcome. The close relationships we form with patients over time open our minds to artistic forms, such as music, that provide valuable emotional support.

I have worked closely with Dr. Nagarsheth and several of his co-authors in caring for patients, and encouraged them as they have sought to incorporate music into our specialty. For many years there were informal gatherings of musically inclined members at the annual meeting of the Society of Gynecologic Oncologists (SGO). In 2001, I was program chair of their annual meeting, and asked my partner Dr. John Soper to lead the first jam session that was a formal part of the meeting agenda. This seemed like a natural fit, since the meeting was held in Nashville – Music City USA.

In 2008 country music gave way to rock and roll. Under the guidance of impresario Dr. G. Larry Maxwell (another former trainee), the N.E.D. band made their debut at the SGO annual meeting in Tampa. In my role as SGO President that year, I had invested heart and soul in planning all aspects of the meeting. The venue was beautiful and the educational and social events rewarding, but as the event has receded in the rearview mirror, the dominant memory that lives on is the awe-inspiring performance of the N.E.D. band. They have followed up this initial success with more music making, awareness raising, and now this amazing book. Silence is dead, long live N.E.D."

Andrew Berchuck, MD
Director, Duke University Division of Gynecologic Oncology
Past-President, Society of Gynecologic Oncologists

Continued on next page

"This is a fascinating book! It is easy to read, well written, and each page leaves you wanting more. Being involved in music my entire life I always sensed the magical healing powers of music, but never before imagined capturing these ideas into words until now. No matter what kind of illness you or your loved ones might be suffering from, *Music and Cancer* will change your life!"

Sweet Georgia Brown
Jazz, Gospel, and R&B Singer

"Part self cancer-care guide, part medical lesson, part music lesson, and part history lesson, *Music and Cancer* rocks. Enjoy, as I did, an unusual duet: how one outstanding surgeon took his passion—the learning, playing, and writing of music—and used it to harmonize communication and the best quality care for his cancer patients and their loved ones. Which is music to my ears baby!"

Fran Drescher
US Public Diplomacy Envoy for Women's Health Issues
Founder and Visionary, Cancer Schmancer Movement
The Nanny

"This is an important book for every patient and their doctors to read. As a cancer doctor and also as a cancer survivor, I appreciate the 'healing' power of music and other nontraditional methods now being used in the treatment of patients with cancer. Not only is Dr. Nagarsheth a great cancer doctor, but also an individual who sees beyond the horizon. He has brought together a talented group of cancer doctors to include music as part of their professional and personal lives. His personal experience with music in his life and career is moving. The book is a testament to the importance of the healing power of music in our lives."

Carolyn D. Runowicz, MD
Past President of the American Cancer Society
Past President of the Society of Gynecologic Oncologists
Chair, National Cancer Advisory Board

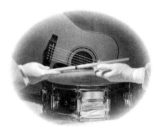

Music
and
Cancer

A Prescription for Healing

Nimesh P. Nagarsheth, MD

Assistant Professor
Division of Gynecologic Oncology
Department of Obstetrics, Gynecology, and
Reproductive Science
Mount Sinai School of Medicine
New York, NY
&
Associate Director of Robotic Surgery
Englewood Hospital and Medical Center
Englewood, NJ

Foreword by **Fran Drescher**

JONES AND BARTLETT PUBLISHERS
Sudbury, Massachusetts
BOSTON   TORONTO   LONDON   SINGAPORE

World Headquarters

Jones and Bartlett Publishers	Jones and Bartlett Publishers	Jones and Bartlett Publishers
40 Tall Pine Drive	Canada	International
Sudbury, MA 01776	6339 Ormindale Way	Barb House, Barb Mews
978-443-5000	Mississauga, Ontario L5V 1J2	London W6 7PA
info@jbpub.com	Canada	United Kingdom
www.jbpub.com		

Jones and Bartlett's books and products are available through most bookstores and online booksellers. To contact Jones and Bartlett Publishers directly, call 800-832-0034, fax 978-443-8000, or visit our website, www.jbpub.com.

Substantial discounts on bulk quantities of Jones and Bartlett's publications are available to corporations, professional associations, and other qualified organizations. For details and specific discount information, contact the special sales department at Jones and Bartlett via the above contact information or send an email to specialsales@jbpub.com.

The authors, editor, and publisher have made every effort to provide accurate information. However, they are not responsible for errors, omissions, or for any outcomes related to the use of the contents of this book and take no responsibility for the use of the products and procedures described. Treatments and side effects described in this book may not be applicable to all people; likewise, some people may require a dose or experience a side effect that is not described herein. Drugs and medical devices are discussed that may have limited availability controlled by the Food and Drug Administration (FDA) for use only in a research study or clinical trial. Research, clinical practice, and government regulations often change the accepted standard in this field. When consideration is being given to use of any drug in the clinical setting, the healthcare provider or reader is responsible for determining FDA status of the drug, reading the package insert, and reviewing prescribing information for the most up-to-date recommendations on dose, precautions, and contraindications, and determining the appropriate usage for the product. This is especially important in the case of drugs that are new or seldom used.

Production Credits

Executive Publisher: Christopher Davis	V.P., Manufacturing and Inventory Control:
Sr. Editorial Assistant: Jessica Acox	Therese Connell
Production Director: Amy Rose	Composition: SNP Best-set Typesetter Ltd., Hong Kong
Production Editor: Daniel Stone	Printing and Binding: Malloy, Inc.
Marketing Manager: Alisha Weisman	Cover Printing: Malloy, Inc.

Cover Credits
Cover Design: Nimesh P. Nagarsheth, MD
Cover Images: Dexter Lane

Library of Congress Cataloging-in-Publication Data
Nagarsheth, Nimesh P.
  Music and cancer : a prescription for healing / Nimesh P. Nagarsheth.
    p. ; cm.
  Includes bibliographical references and index.
  ISBN-13: 978-0-7637-7908-5
  ISBN-10: 0-7637-7908-3
  1. Cancer. 2. Music therapy. 3. Music. I. Title.
  [DNLM: 1. Neoplasms–psychology. 2. Neoplasms–therapy. 3. Music
Therapy. 4. Music. 5. Patient Education as Topic. QZ 266 N147m 2010]
  RC254.5.N34 2010
  616.99′406–dc22
                              2009019550

6048

Printed in the United States of America
13 12 11 10 09   10 9 8 7 6 5 4 3 2 1

Dedication

To my amazing parents; my supportive brother,
Shailesh, and sister-in-law, Monika; my beautiful niece,
Alisha, and nephew, Aidan; and my incredible patients—
all of you have shown me the truth of life.

CONTENTS

Music is the pulse of life.
It's the gift that keeps on giving,
and musicians are a blessing in our lives.

Ovarian Cancer Survivor
Brooklyn, NY

John F. Boggess, MD
Associate Professor
Director, Robotic Assisted Medicine Center
Division of Gynecology Oncology
University of North Carolina
Chapel Hill, NC
   [Member N.E.D., Guitar, Lead Vocals]

K.J. Denhert
Recording Artist, Motéma Music
New York, NY

Frank Forte, MD
Dizzy Gillespie Cancer Institute
Englewood Hospital and Medical Center
Englewood, NJ

Jana Herzen
President, Motéma Music
New York, NY

Joanie M. Hope, MD
Fellow, Gynecologic Oncology
New York University Medical Center
New York, NY
   [Member N.E.D., Lead Vocals, Guitar]

James H. Latimer
Professor Emeritus, School of Music
University of Wisconsin–Madison
Madison, WI

Tony Martell
Chairman and Founder, T.J. Martell Foundation
New York, NY

Arden Moulton, LMSW
Woman to Woman Program Coordinator
Department of Social Work Services
Mount Sinai Medical Center
New York, NY

William "Rusty" Robinson, MD
Professor, Director of Clinical Research
Harrington Cancer Center
Texas Tech University Health Science Center
Amarillo, TX
 [Member N.E.D., Bass Guitar, Harmonica, Vocals]

John T. Soper, MD
The Hendricks Professor of Obstetrics and Gynecology
Division of Gynecologic Oncology
University of North Carolina
Chapel Hill, NC
 [Member N.E.D., Guitar]

Ken Trush
Co-Founder, Daniel's Music Foundation
New York, NY

William E. Winter, III, MD
Northwest Cancer Specialists
Portland, OR
 [Member N.E.D., Lead Guitar]

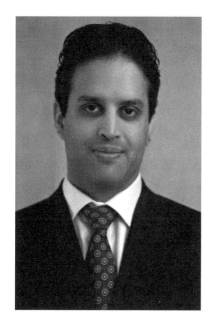

Photo by Dexter Lane.

Nimesh P. Nagarsheth, MD, is a gynecologic oncologist and has a busy clinical practice at Mount Sinai Medical Center (New York, NY) and Englewood Hospital and Medical Center (Englewood, NJ). Dr. Nagarsheth is a member of the faculty at the Mount Sinai School of Medicine and is also actively involved in teaching and performing cutting-edge research. In his practice, Dr. Nagarsheth provides the full range of surgical and medical gynecologic oncology care. His specialized interests include cancer prevention, advanced radical laparoscopic surgery, including robotic surgery, and novel approaches to cancer management. He has numerous publications and is a leading author in several landmark medical research studies. Dr. Nagarsheth has developed an extensive background in blood management in the field of gynecologic oncology and is considered one of the world's experts in performing bloodless (transfusion-free) cancer surgery. A frequent speaker at national meetings, he has received a number of teaching and research awards.

Dr. Nagarsheth earned his bachelor's degree from the University of Wisconsin–Madison and his medical degree from the Mount Sinai

School of Medicine. He completed his residency training in obstetrics and gynecology at Duke University Medical Center, and his fellowship training in gynecologic oncology at Mount Sinai. During this training, Dr. Nagarsheth also conducted important research projects at New York University Medical Center and Memorial Sloan-Kettering Cancer Center in New York.

In addition to his career as a surgeon, Dr. Nagarsheth is an accomplished musician and currently plays drums and percussion, keyboards, and guitar for several bands. In 2008, Dr. Nagarsheth and five of his medical colleagues from around the country founded the rock band N.E.D., an acronym for No Evidence of Disease. Following their first show at the Tampa Convention Center (Tampa, FL), N.E.D. received an invitation to play at the first ever Gynecologic Cancer Awareness Movement (GCAM) in Washington, DC in November 2009. Bringing together political leaders, physicians and caregivers, researchers, advocacy groups, and of course patients from around the world, GCAM sparked the interest for N.E.D. to define a meaningful purpose and mission for the band in raising awareness for gynecologic cancers. In 2008, N.E.D. was signed onto the New York City-based record label Motéma Music with a concept to help promote gynecologic cancer awareness, education, research, and fundraising through their music. Since that time, N.E.D. has been invited to play throughout the United States and internationally, and continues to develop and shape the role of music in the healing process.

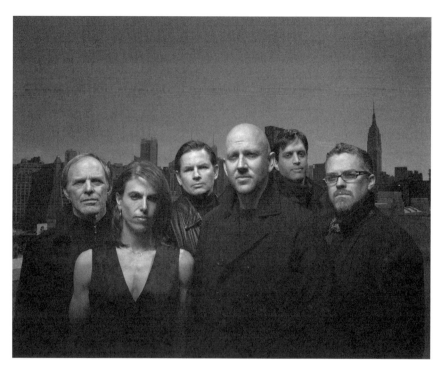

N.E.D. members are (from left to right) doctors John T. Soper, Joanie M. Hope, Rusty Robinson, John F. Boggess, Nimesh P. Nagarsheth, and William E. Winter.
Photo by Craig LaCourt.

by Fran Drescher

You're probably sitting there wondering, "What in the hell does Fran Drescher know about music or cancer? Isn't she *The Nanny* with the nasal voice and funny laugh?"

Sure that's all true. But I have news for you, my friend; I'm also a cancer survivor. During the last season of *The Nanny* I was experiencing symptoms. Little did I know I was about to embark upon a two-year, eight-doctor odyssey in search of a proper diagnosis of uterine cancer. Honey, I got in the stirrups more times than Roy Rogers!

I didn't bother to question my doctors when they said that I was too young for cancer. Frankly, I was so glad to still be too young for anything! But all the while I continued to be misdiagnosed and mistreated for a peri-menopausal condition I didn't have. If only I knew then what I know now!

Nine years later, *The Nanny* continues to be on the air alive and well around the world and so am I. Even better, I've found ways to turn my pain into purpose and lemons into lemonade. First by writing what became a New York Times best-seller, *Cancer Schmancer*; next founding the Cancer Schmancer Movement, a not-for-profit organization dedicated to ensuring Stage 1 diagnosis, when cancer is most curable, for all women with cancer; and most recently by being appointed as the Public Diplomacy Envoy for Women's Health Issues at The US State Department. Sometimes the best gifts come in the ugliest packages . . .

You can imagine why, as an actress turned women's health advocate, I was immediately drawn to the gynecologic oncologists rock band called No Evidence of Disease (N.E.D.), when my colleague, Dr. G. Larry Maxwell, Head of Gynecologic Oncology at Walter Reed Army Medical Center, brought them to my attention. It's not too often that you find people in this world who have equal passions for both art and science, and far fewer who find ways to tie them together in one neat bow.

I consider myself lucky to have crossed paths with Dr. Nagarsheth, the author of this mind-expanding book. Because, like me, he and his other doctor band members are as passionate about fighting cancer as they are about creating meaningful art.

As if saving the lives of patients with cancer and producing an album with his rock band weren't enough, he had to go and write a book about it. So, of course, I had to read it. And, I'm thrilled that you're joining me on this journey through music and cancer, too. It was Chapter 7 that really blew my mind. Dr. Nagarsheth hit the nail on the head when he used the woodblock example, a simple musical exercise, as a metaphor to describe just how a doctor and patient should engage with one another during an appointment. In the exercise, you have the music student holding a steady rhythm while the teacher plays another rhythm. Sounds easy enough, but it takes special skill to have two instruments playing two rhythms at one time in harmony. What does this have to do with cancer? Let me tell you, if I had been a medical consumer back then, I would have had the skills to harmonize with my doctors and maintain my own rhythm instead of getting all caught up in theirs!

If you ever think your body's trying to tell you something's wrong, listen to it. Cancer at its earliest and most curable stages comes in whispers. Find your rhythm and don't go losing it the second you walk through the doctor's office doors. Sure you're scared and those white coats can be intimidating, but you know your body best and don't you forget it. Speak up, be specific, listen closely for a response and ask questions when you need help making sense of it all. As Dr. Nagarsheth cleverly points out, for doctors, musical listening focuses awareness on both sides of the story—on one side are the patient's fears, needs, and questions, and on the other side is the doctor's own desire to provide the best, most appropriate care. Transform from being a patient into a medical consumer. Become better partners with your physician because it can save your life. Take control of your body!

Part self cancer-care guide, part medical lesson, part music lesson, and part history lesson, *Music and Cancer* rocks. Enjoy, as I did, an unusual duet: how one outstanding surgeon took his passion—the learning, playing, and writing of music—and used it to harmonize communication and the best quality care for his cancer patients and their loved ones. Which is music to my ears baby!

Be well,

Fran Drescher
U.S. Public Diplomacy Envoy for Women's Health Issues
Founder and Visionary, Cancer Schmancer Movement
The Nanny

I never grew up wanting to be a doctor. There are no doctors in my immediate family and my childhood interactions with the medical profession were limited to just a few emergency room visits, the occasional vaccination, and other routine health maintenance exams. Music was my passion in my youth. I grew up wanting to be a rock star!

In fourth grade, I had my first drum lesson. Why drums? Because my older brother had already given up the violin and keyboards and as such, my dad did not expect me to seriously pursue any instrument over the long-term. Drums, which require only a rubber practice pad, two sticks, and some sheet music, seemed like the most inexpensive investment for this likely short-lived endeavor. However, as the lessons began, my fascination with music became stronger.

Like a lot of kids growing up in suburban America, I always struggled to fit in. Facing peer pressure and the uncertainties of youth, I leaned on music to get me through it all. Music was my out, my escape from reality. Even at a young age, I realized the power of music and the magic it created. Then, one Friday night during the sixth grade, my life was transformed. My older brother and his friend had plans to see a rock concert in New Haven, but, as fate would have it, the concert was postponed because the singer became ill. The concert date was moved from earlier in the week to that Friday and my brother's friend was no longer able to attend due to a family conflict. When my brother asked our dad what to do regarding the extra ticket, he responded simply "take your brother." And so it was, without any input on the matter, I was commissioned to attend the Rush concert at the New Haven Coliseum. This was my first rock concert, and I was terrified. Images of black leather jackets stampeding the stage ran through my head. How would I survive? Suffice it to say the concert was not as I had imagined it would be at all. The crowd was entranced in the music and the performers, and I realized it was simply all about the music. The concert was amazing. I had just seen some of the most skillful and talented musicians of our time, and their art left a lasting impression. That night I identified my childhood hero: Neil Peart, drummer, percussionist, and lyricist from Rush.

Everyone has a childhood hero, someone they aspire to be like and look up to. Whether a family member, celebrity, or other role model, having someone you can identify with can be a precious part of growing up. Sometimes childhood heroes disappoint society, such as the occasional athlete or musician who gets involved with drugs or other illegal activity. It is a great responsibility to be a hero, and hopefully your own childhood hero was always a positive influence on you.

Neil Peart is one of the most respected drummers in the world. I have followed his career closely over the years and can attest that his talent is the result of discipline and hard work. He is widely respected in the music community and is well known not only in the rock genre of music but also in areas such as African music and jazz. In 2008, he directed the Buddy Rich Memorial Concert in New York City (Buddy Rich is the most famous jazz drummer ever to have played in the history of jazz). For the jazz community to pick a rock drummer to run the Buddy Rich Memorial Concert is one of the most telling signs of his success as a modern-day drummer.

You may be asking yourself how the story of Neil Peart is pertinent to the preface of this book. Neil suffered tragedies beyond imagination, losing his entire immediate family over the course of 1 year. His 19-year-old daughter died in a car accident, and 10 months later his wife died of "terminal cancer." I have no further informa-tion on the specifics of his wife's cancer except that it seemed like maintaining a good quality of life was near impossible given the loss of her daughter just a few months prior. Please do not interpret this story to mean that everyone with cancer dies from cancer. This, of course, is not true, and is not the point of mentioning this story. Neil has written about his tragedies and his healing process in his book entitled, *Ghost Rider: Travels on the Healing Road.*

I was a second-year resident in obstetrics and gynecology at Duke University Medical Center in North Carolina when I heard of Neil's double tragedy, and my heart sank thinking of the suffering that he must have experienced. Neil did recover and five years later Rush re-emerged as a successful rock band on the music scene. His story and his incredible recovery from these events has been a great source of inspiration for his many fans, including me. Anytime I feel that my problems in my life are overwhelming, I remember his story and the many more equally inspiring stories that I have witnessed taking care of cancer patients in my current role as a practicing cancer surgeon in New York City. Life truly is beautiful.

Working with cancer patients has been the most rewarding experience of my life, and I hope to continue to fight cancer and improve the quality of life of cancer patients for as long as I am physically able. While advances in research and medical care seem to be growing at an exponential rate, advances in the improvement of the quality of life have not been a priority until recently. This may be due to the common misconception that quality of life does not have a scientifically measurable impact on a patient's outcome. In this book, we explore the role of music on cancer healing in an effort to help improve the quality of life of cancer patients. Through this artistic approach, we hope to touch the reader in a way that could not be accomplished from a traditional medical practice. With the help of musicians, physicians, and patients, we have collected some of the most inspiring examples that have touched our lives. We hope that you will be able to identify with these examples and discover how beautiful life truly is. Cancer or not, we are all in this together.

Nimesh P. Nagarsheth, MD

ACKNOWLEDGMENTS

I thank my parents, my brother Shailesh and sister-in-law Monika, and my niece Alisha and nephew Aidan for the incredible support and encouragement they have provided me with over my lifetime, especially in the past year and a half during my work on the N.E.D. project.

I also thank my fellow N.E.D. members (doctors John Boggess, Joanie Hope, John Soper, Rusty Robinson, and William Winter) for their friendship, support, and wonderful contributions to this book. In addition, I would like to thank everyone who has participated and continues to believe in the N.E.D. collaboration, including Dr. G. Larry Maxwell, the group at Motéma Music (Jana Herzen, K.J. Denhert, Mario McNulty, and friends), the group at Jones and Bartlett Publishing (Chris Davis, Kathy Richardson, Jessica Acox, Daniel Stone, Barb Bartoszek), the Gynecologic Cancer Foundation (Karen Carlson, Marsha Wilson, and friends), Carol Berman (City Girl Media), Wendy Oxenhorn (Jazz Foundation of America), Robert Friedman (Radical Media), Dr. Jim Holland, Tony Martell (T.J. Martell Foundation), and Fran Drescher and her group at Cancer Schmancer (Erika Strauss, Laurie Meadoff, and Shikha Vasaiwala).

From my department and division, I thank my mentors, doctors Michael Brodman, Peter Dottino, Carmel Cohen, and Jamal Rahaman as well as all of my partners and colleagues (especially Arden Moulton) at Mount Sinai Medical Center for their guidance, inspiration, and continued support in my academic career in medicine. I send out a special thanks to Dr. Carolyn Runowicz for her encouragement during this project.

I thank the outstanding physicians and staff (especially my colleagues, the operating room staff, and the office staff) at Englewood

Hospital and Medical Center for the world-class care they provide for my patients and unwavering support for this book. A special thanks goes to Dr. Frank Forte and the entire medical oncology division for always believing in me and helping to make this book a reality.

For his friendship, dedication, and countless hours of editing, I appreciate the help of Nitin Chopra (who, at this writing, is single in NYC). For contributions in photography, I would like to thank Dexter Lane (courtesy of Peter Arnold), Barbara Niss (Mount Sinai Archives), Sandra Sgambati (Englewood Hospital), Craig LaCourt, and Claudia Robinson.

Finally, for his lifetime of mentorship and for sharing with me the secret of life, I would like to thank Professor Jim Latimer. And for their strength, courage, wisdom, compassion, and love, I thank my amazing patients.

Nimesh P. Nagarsheth, MD

From the Top

Nimesh P. Nagarsheth, MD

"Alright, let's take it from the top. Remember, it's not as difficult as you think. If it will help you, think of it as a scientific graph in chemistry class where you have points on the vertical axis and horizontal axis, which provide you with information that you have to constantly interpret and react to. Reading music is no different than reading that scientific graph. Okay, ready and . . .".

And that is how it all began—a simple observation between playing a piece of music and life as a college student. I was in my freshman year of college at the University of Wisconsin in Madison and was majoring in zoology. But my true love was music. Even at a young age I felt the power of music and the amazing possibilities that one could achieve through this form of expression. I had been studying and playing the drums since elementary school and bought my first drum set while in junior high school. I continued drumming throughout high school and played in several bands from jazz to rock to hard core. I thought I knew what music was all about. But it wasn't until I reached college that I realized my knowledge was only the tip of the iceberg (a very large iceberg).

Professor Jim Latimer was head of the percussion department at the University of Wisconsin when I began college. He is a world-class percussionist with an incredible understanding of music and an outstanding reputation for performance as well as teaching. It wasn't long before I managed to convince him to take me on as his student, which consisted of weekly 1-hour lessons in the percussion studio.

The studio held all the wonders of the percussion world including marimbas, vibraphones, drums and cymbals of all shapes and sizes, and a variety of other percussion instruments. Each lesson was divided into the following four parts: sight-reading studies, repertoire studies, improvisation studies, and exploratory studies. Sight-reading studies consisted of playing a new piece of music on the spot without any preparation, and repertoire studies consisted of playing a piece of music that I had been preparing during the previous week. Improvisation studies focused on exchanging solos on the drum set or marimba, and exploratory studies focused on becoming comfortable with unfamiliar territories such as chord structures and scales that may be considered outside the box.

I continued lessons with Professor Latimer throughout my college years, and by the time I graduated we had developed a friendship that would bond us for life. Nine years later, I was a fully trained obstetrician and gynecologist receiving specialized training in gynecologic oncology at the Mount Sinai Medical Center in New York City. It was then, just 6 weeks after the September 11th tragedy shook New York City, when I decided to take a weekend escape back to my college roots in Wisconsin, which included a visit with Professor Latimer (now retired on a farm just outside Madison).

The farm house and the newly-built adjoining music studio (complete with marimbas, drum set, and various other percussion instruments) provided the ideal setting for the reunion of the student and teacher. With ice cubes clinking, the catching up and the exchange of information began. We each had so much to say—so much had happened. As he showed me the latest musical arrangements he had been working on for the Madison Marimba Quartet, I showed him the recent instructional video I had made demonstrating the techniques of radical cancer surgery at the Mount Sinai Medical Center. He was thrilled to discover that I had applied music from the Madison Marimba Quartet as background music for the video. Then the time had come for another lesson and jam session in the studio. Ideas were flowing freely and spirits were high, and as we played into the night and let the music carry us away to another place, together we discovered it. Quite possibly music was the key to unlocking the secrets of life, and that everything we do in life is reflected in music. More importantly, we realized that a better understanding of music may lead to a better understanding of life.

Eight years have passed since that unforgettable weekend getaway, and I still think about the revelation we had relating music and life. My medical training has completed, and I now have a busy career as a cancer surgeon in New York City specializing in gynecologic oncology. Working with cancer patients has been the most rewarding experience in my life and the motivation for me to constantly search for better ways to help my patients mentally and physically win the fight against cancer.

And then I made the connection! Music is that magical tool I have been looking for. Using the concepts learned in music, I have been able to (both consciously and unconsciously) improve the quality of life of my patients. Soon, I met other gynecologic oncologists from around the country who shared my love for music and had made this same connection with their patients. We quickly realized that our story needed to be told and thus, *Music and Cancer* was born. We have combined our vastly different experiences to form a new understanding of cancer healing and would like to share these ideas with you.

As we take you through the wonders of music as it relates to every-day experiences, we hope that you will make the incredible discovery that we (and our patients) have made.

PART I

The Evolving Relationship Between Music and Medicine

CHAPTER 1

Tuning Up

Music—Older than Written History— As Young as Tomorrow

James H. Latimer and Nimesh P. Nagarsheth, MD

We realize that many of you may currently be in the fight of your life battling cancer and that you may have questions that urgently need to be addressed. For some of you, the diagnosis is relatively recent, and many unanswered questions remain about initial treatment options and the road ahead. For others, new challenges may arise and questions regarding the recurrence or progression of your disease may be your primary concern. Still others of you may be in a state of remission, which is also known as no evidence of disease (N.E.D.), and remain hopeful for a cure during your time of close surveillance.

Regardless of where you may be in the cancer process, we would like to help you. Unfortunately, this book will not cure cancer, nor will it answer all of your burning questions regarding cancer prevention, diagnosis, and treatment. However, this book may improve your quality of life by helping you understand the disease process through a more artistic (and therefore more humanistic) approach.

Music is the medium we have chosen to help explore these humanistic concepts. Because everyone has a different background and appreciation for music, we believed that the best starting point would be to briefly review the history of music. Understanding the evolution of music from its origins to modern music is critical to the premise of this book, and provides the foundation for the chapters that follow. Therefore, before delving into the relationships and parallels between music and cancer healing, we ask that you indulge us for a short diversion from the daily stresses of life and join us on this fascinating journey through the history of music. Just as a musician must take the time to tune his instrument before playing in order to get the most out of his performance, think of this as your time to tune up on the history of music before you start the big show.

On the wall of the Latimer Music Studio, running across the drop ceiling is a sign with the adage: "Older than written history–as young as tomorrow." Although this refers to the musical art of percussion, it could just as well refer to music. The history of music as we know it is older than written history. We have what we often call the periods of music: prehistoric, ancient, early, medieval, renaissance, baroque, classical, romantic, 20th century, and 21st century.

Prehistoric, ancient, and much of the early music is not written. We most often associate prehistoric with the music in Europe before the development of writing. True prehistoric may well be that of traditional, indigenous, or folk music—music that to this day is not written including African, Native American, and American jazz. Traditional or folk music is cultural. Each group had their own tradition.

Early and medieval music is often described as early church or church-type music for out of it came the long tradition of Gregorian chant because the Roman Catholic church did much to preserve and control musical development during this time. There is often an overlap of reference to early music right on through the Medieval, Renaissance, and Baroque periods. So as not to bore you with the facts, we are reminded of really great books already published on the history of music, from the 10-volume *Grove's Dictionary of Music* to David Barber's *If it Ain't Baroque* and *Bach, Beethoven, and the Boys.* The latter two books take you through the Baroque, Classical, and Romantic periods of music subtitled, "music history as it should have been taught." Of course, there are many notable books on the history of music and these are available at your local bookstore or library. Some of the greatest music of all time has come from the Baroque, Classical, and Romantic periods of music. These include the likes of Haydn, Handel, Bach, Beethoven, Brahms, and a host of others.

This brings us to the 20th century of music, music writing, performance, and interpretation. In this country, the development of the percussion family of instruments as a performance art is 20th century. It is interesting to note that in one of his documentaries, George Paige shows the particular mating stories of different species, among them, the Palm cockatoo. The history of percussion as a tool (performance art) begins with this age-old bird. By instinct, this cockatoo breaks off a twig of a certain diameter, puts it in his mouth and flies to the highest hollowed out dead tree. Once perched, the cockatoo retrieves the stick and, with the thickest end, begins to tap rhythmically on the more hollow part of the dead tree. He has his own drum and uses it to signal for a mate. Western percussion may have developed as a performance art in the 20th century, but the bird had it as its mating call perhaps since the beginning of time.

Calling is an early use of music. Think about the cowbell, Swiss alpenhorn, and the military drum. In all of the early wars of the Americas, drummers accompanied the troops to signal and give messages. Native Americans had traditional or folk rituals of song and dance using the drum for all of life's happenings from birth to death, peace and war, prayer and honor, and so on.

The advent of technology from the Edison phonograph to the victrola and glass records, to vinyl records, and stereos to television, to beta and 8-track, cassettes to CDs, DVDs to iPods and iPhones, and home theaters, the 20th century music escalated beyond all expectations. Who said we could not fly to the moon? Twentieth century music was born. Twentieth century music unveiled American jazz, which grew out of the ancient or traditional, unwritten, folk kind of music. It is the people's music. From Africa via American jazz came the varieties of music we now call blues, hip-hop, popular, rock and roll, hard rock, and rap. The latter is so exciting that we now have the "Rappin' Mathematician," who has found it an easy way for kids to love and to learn math. Of their teacher, these kids say, "he's cool." Remember the roaring 1920s when the Charleston dance style reigned? Follow this with the jitterbug of the 1930s and the 1940s, the genius of Ray Charles, and the legacy and inspiration of Duke Ellington. Remember what happened when Elvis, who looked like he was put together with a string, sang "Ain't Nothin' But a Hound Dog?" Remember the 60s and what happened one cool evening on the Ed Sullivan show? The Beatles came to America. America has not been the same since. The world has not been the same since. They were followed by a host of young artists who began to experiment with music and with technology. When the people's Princess died, it was Elton John who said it all in his moving tribute, "Candle in the Wind." Who would have ever thought the day is here when we have Presidents of the United States using songs as their themes (President William Jefferson Clinton "Don't Stop Thinkin' About Tomorrow" by Christine McVie and President Barack H. Obama using "Signed, Sealed, Delivered, I'm Yours" by Stevie Wonder). In fact, in July 2008, then President-elect Obama had the German rock band Reamonn warm up a crowd of 200,000 people at Victory Column in Berlin just before his speech. Needless to say, he received a rock star type welcome and had a fired up crowd eager to hear his speech. After the show, Obama became an honorary member of Reamonn after the leader of the band gave him one of only five band rings that were ever made.

Today we are continuing to explore new musical avenues and push the envelope on inspiration. N.E.D. is the cancer patient's band. With six musician cancer surgeons incorporating all the styles that have influenced them to make music of the 21st century, N.E.D. is more than a band. N.E.D. is a musical tool to inform, involve, and instruct others about the prevention and cures for cancer.

In all of this, the basic ingredients of music remain the same: melody, rhythm, harmony, and form. Music calls. It beckons, it heals, and it soothes. Music of the ages is used as a messenger. What is "music" to someone's ears may not be the same music to another person. Of music, it can be said that it is rhythm (motion) in sound. From the cockatoo tapping on the dead tree and sounding his love message to potential mates to six modern day surgeons bridging the gap between medicine and music, music is older than written history and as young as tomorrow.

CHAPTER 2

Music as a Science, Medicine as an Art

Nimesh P. Nagarsheth, MD

Music is as much a science as medicine is an art. Personally, I like to think of art and science balanced on a scale much like two kids playing on a seesaw. Although music falls closer to the art side and medicine falls closer to the science side, both possess forces that influence the entire length of the scale and therefore significantly overlap. At times, the scale will tip towards one side or the other, but the forces of art and science in life always find a way to balance each other out. This is because in life, science cannot survive without art, and art cannot survive without science. Just as you need two kids to keep the ends of the seesaw moving up and down, both music and medicine thrive on a dynamic balance of science and art (**Figure 2-1**).

For the scientific scholars out there who may have difficulty believing that an art form such as music could have any relationship to science and medicine, I understand your reservations. However, stick with me and I will do my best to convince you otherwise.

First, at its foundation, written music is based on notes and rests. This language of music is universal, and serves to transfer information from performer to performer, and performer to listener. Even across vastly different cultures and languages, the reproducibility of written music is universal and allows for the exchange of ideas

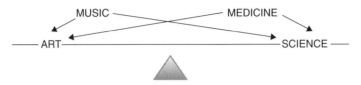

Figure 2-1. A graphical representation of the balance between art and science as it relates to the fields of music and medicine.

between cultures in a unique fashion. Furthermore, written music is precise and exacting, and each note designates a specific tone and duration of time that the performer will play. The first description of the mathematical exactness of the tone of musical notes comes from the Greek philosopher Pythagoras somewhere around the time of 500 BC. Pythagoras and his followers were experts in both mathematics and music, and therefore were well positioned to make this connection. Through his works and observations, he found that the tone of a note produced by hitting a piece of string was directly dependent on its length. Expanding on this discovery, Pythagoras realized that musical notes or tones could be given a numerical value, and that the musical scale of notes corresponded to an exact, reproducible progression of numbers. He believed that a better understanding of the universe could be obtained through the integration of music and science, and postulated the concept of the Harmony of the Spheres, which he referred to as the music of nature. The Harmony of the Spheres is music heard in the mind (not audible) as a result of an interpretation based on the comparison of proportions and distances of the planets and stars to the numerical progression of the musical scale. Although a somewhat difficult concept to grasp, the Harmony of the Spheres represents the complete integration of music and science within the human mind.

Modern day Pythagoreans are among us. If you ever get a chance to spend some time with one of them, it can be an eye-opening experience. During my college years, I concentrated my studies on both music and science, and spent several hours a week working in a scientific laboratory next to the office of a famous zoologist, whom

I will refer to as Dr. Smith. Although I passed by Dr. Smith several times a day walking the halls, I never actually interacted with him in the school of sciences. Instead, I got to know him during a percussion clinic he conducted in the school of music. This was not surprising to me as he was well-known around campus for his scientific accomplishments as well as for his extraordinary piano playing skills. In fact, he had the reputation for playing music like a machine. This is not to say his music lacked heart or emotion; it's just that his style was exacting and allowed no room for error. His groove was tightly on the beat (otherwise known as *burying the beat*; described in Chapter 14). Every note was intentional and his performance was precise. Watching him play, it was clear that his accomplished musical abilities were rooted in the fundamentals of hard work and discipline (in contrast to the creative musical talent that some individuals seem to be born with). One of Dr. Smith's favorite and most interesting demonstrations (a scientific experiment of sorts) involved taking phone numbers from members of the audience at random and transcribing this information into a melody for an original piece of music that he would compose on the spot. When I asked him how he was able to do this so accurately and smoothly, he quickly explained that he considers musical notes in terms of a numeric value and vice versa. He went on to state that when he needed to remember a sequence of numbers in his daily life (for example, when conducting experiments in the lab), he wouldn't memorize the numbers directly, but instead would memorize the melody these numbers represented. When the time came to recall these numbers, he simply would hum the melody and would then be able to translate this information back to the original sequence of numbers. Whether or not he knew it, this scientific guru was definitely a modern day Pythagorean. In stark contrast to the artistry with which I had normally associated music, I now had my first hands-on experience of how music is fundamentally derived directly from the principles of math and science.

The ability of the human mind to integrate the fields of music and science is actually not as far-fetched as you may think. Consider the fact that music at its core represents the process of measuring and deciding. In other words, a musician playing a piece of music is constantly reacting to, evaluating, and interpreting events in the environment. These events may take the form of notes on a sheet of music or simply positive or negative energy derived from one's emotions or feelings. The performer must measure this information (decipher what is important and what is extraneous) and decide how to present it to the listener in a way that he or she believes to be its most truthful and purest form. Listeners will then have the final say as to whether they believe in the musician's proposal (i.e., they like the music), or reject the musician's proposal (they are not a fan of the music). Does this sound familiar? It is actually very similar to the scientific method that has been used throughout the centuries to advance science. This method is a powerful tool that basically is a stepwise approach to reaching the truth. It involves making observations, formulating a hypothesis, testing the hypothesis (measuring), and reaching a conclusion about the truth (deciding). In this light, both music and science represent a quest for the truth through the same fundamental virtues of measuring and deciding.

Interlude

Although it would be nice to think of music purely as a truthful art form, music has been victim to the darker side of humanity and has suffered from greed, deceit, manipulation of facts, and creation of falsehoods throughout history. Probably one of the most infamous examples of this in contemporary times centers on the rise and fall of the music group Milli Vanilli. This pop group became extremely popular in the late 1980s largely based on the success of a few songs including the hit "Girl You Know It's True." In 1989, during a live performance in Bristol, Connecticut, the singers ran into a problem when it was discovered (through a glitch in some prerecorded music) that the singers on stage were not actually singing the song. Word quickly spread that the two front men in Milli Vanilli were falsely credited for singing songs that were not their own. After a series of complaints and concerns from the public and the media, Milli Vanilli's Grammy Award was rescinded and the record company permanently deleted their album from their music catalog. Even something as beautiful and innocent as music must continuously strive to remain true to its art form.

Professor Latimer is also a strong believer in the relationship between music and science, and through my weekly lessons in his studio, I was able to learn how to apply this knowledge in everyday life. In fact, a quote from Professor Latimer taken from one of my very first lessons (an excerpt from the first paragraph of this book) was the inspiration for me to begin exploring the relationships between music and other aspects of life. During this lesson, in response to my frustration regarding difficulty I had reading a piece of music, Professor Latimer stated, "Think of it as a scientific graph in chemistry class where you have points on the vertical axis and horizontal axis, which provide you with information that you have to constantly interpret and react to. Reading music is no different than reading that scientific graph." Suddenly, with this new mindset, I was able to read the piece of music and played the part flawlessly. It was as if I had learned the secret of music. I realized that performing music did not need to be a struggle, as it was just a reflection of things that we do in everyday life (reading, writing, measuring, and deciding). And as such, music is as natural as science.

A Working Example of the Relationship Between the Scientific Graph and Music

In our own little experiment, we wanted to see what an electrocardiogram (ECG) would look like if it were transcribed as written music. The ECG is a graphical representation of the electrical activity of the heart, and provides important information about its mechanical function, structure, and electrical conduction. In **Figure 2-2**, on the left side is an ECG from a patient with hyperkalemia (a potentially life-threatening condition in which the patient has extremely high levels of potassium in the blood). On the right side is what this condition looks like as written music. Without any knowledge of the disease process or background in ECG interpretation, one can imagine the sense of urgency this medical condition possesses through the very noticeable dramatic and sharply pointed peaks. When the written music interpretation of this ECG is played on an instrument, the attacking notes and dramatic pitch changes actually portrays a sense of urgency to the listener. But most importantly, this dramatic musical phrase reminds us of the humanistic process that is taking place beyond this piece of paper. That is, this ECG represents something much more than a textbook graphic example of the medical condition called hyperkalemia. This ECG represents a person who needs immediate attention and medical care.

Making the discovery of the scientific nature of music has definitely been one of the turning points in my life, and has ignited both my artistic and scientific passion for bridging the gap between music and medicine. In my mind, these two fields are connected, and as a physician I am reminded of Professor Latimer's quote every day when interpreting important data related to patient care. Acquiring this knowledge has helped me achieve the ideal balance of science and art in my surgical practice and in my life.

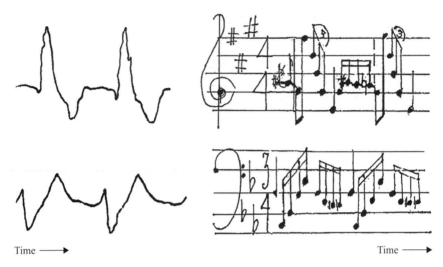

Time ⟶   Time ⟶

Figure 2-2. The left side of this figure demonstrates an ECG of a patient who is experiencing hyperkalemia, which is a potentially life-threatening process that indicates toxic levels of potassium in the blood stream. The right side of this figure demonstrates the musical interpretation of this process as transcribed in written music.

For years, physicians and scientists alike have made several important advances in medicine based on the scientific nature of music. For example, would you be surprised if I told you that the person who invented the stethoscope was a keen musician? In 1816, the French physician Rene Laennec found himself in a difficult situation. Wanting to help a relatively overweight female patient, he needed a way to hear her heart and lungs while respecting her personal boundaries. Prior to the invention of the stethoscope, doctors used a less than sophisticated technique called *direct auscultation*, which basically involved putting an ear on the patient's chest. Calling on his musical background, Laennec improvised and rolled several sheets of paper into a cylinder and put one end to his ear and the other end to the patient's chest. Using this new technique, he discovered that he could hear the patient's heart sounds more clearly and louder than ever before. He formalized his invention and named it "Le Cylindre," which was the first version of the stethoscope. Laennec went on to publish his findings correlating abnormal heart sounds with specific heart and lung diseases, and was the first person to suggest the utility of the stethoscope in the bedside care of patients. Of course, the stethoscope has undergone several major improvements, and today it is best recognized in its polyvinyl chloride tubing binaural form (rubber-like tubing with two ear pieces), instead of the original monaural form (one ear piece) (Figure 2-3). One million stethoscopes are sold annually throughout the world, and they come in all shapes and sizes ranging from those designed to examine the highly specialized cardiology patient to the extremely small pediatric and infant patients. Interestingly, the future of the stethoscope will likely rely even further on the scientific basis of sound through the use of ultrasound technology and imaging, which will provide a more objective way to hear and also visualize the heart at the bedside.

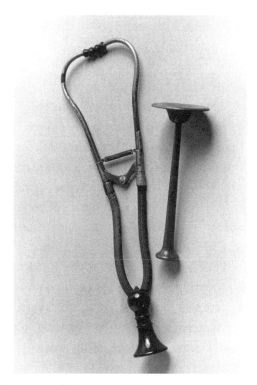

Figure 2-3. Early versions of the monaural (one ear piece) and binaural (two ear pieces) stethoscopes.
Courtesy of the Mount Sinai Archives, New York, NY.

As Laennac eloquently demonstrated, in addition to being a form of entertainment, music can teach us practical uses of the science of sound. By definition, sound (as heard by humans) is simply vibrations that are transmitted through mediums such as a liquid, solid, or gas. Through studying the principles of sound and more specifically ultrasound (vibrations that occur at a higher frequency than what is audible to humans), scientists have found several practical uses for vibration frequency technology in modern medicine. For example, ultrasound imaging is one of the most widely used methods to safely visualize anatomy inside the living human body. From obstetrics to cardiology to cancer, ultrasound imaging has been extremely important in improving the care of patients throughout the world. Incredibly, scientists and engineers also have found ways to harness ultrasonic energy to create operating room instruments. For example, surgical instruments that convert ultrasonic vibrations to mechanical movements are often used in the removal and destruction of cancer during surgery.

Although science is responsible for some amazing advances in medicine, science also has its limitations especially when it comes to medical applications. Returning to our ECG example above, it is worth noting that from a scientific standpoint, modern ECG machines have built-in programs that can interpret ECGs with a great deal of accuracy. These interpretations are often printed at the top of the ECG and inform the physician of potential structural and conduction heart abnormalities that the patient might be suffering. While these machines can diagnose almost any heart condition, they lack the ability to actually treat the patient. This is because the heart does not exist in isolation but of course is part of the incredibly complex human body. As such, treatment of a heart condition must be considered in the context of treatment of the whole person. Regardless of how advanced medicine becomes, therefore, the human touch of the physician will always have an essential role in the care of patients. The ECG represents the quintessential example of the limitation of science in medicine. Simply stated, science without art is like a brain without a "heart."

Although music as a science may be a difficult concept to grasp for many (especially for the non-musician), medicine as an art form seems to be a more generally accepted concept. As a brief introduction to this topic, the importance of art in medicine has been well-described throughout history by a number of prominent medical caregivers. One such scholar was Sir William Withey Gull, an English physician who became famous when caring for the Prince of Wales during his time of illness in the late 1800s. Sir William Gull addressed the importance of incorporating both art and science as a practicing physician and is well-known for the following quote.

"Medicine requires not only the intellectual cultivation of a science, but the patience and the practical skill of an art. At the bedside we must be animated by the feeling of faithful artisans, of men whose object and duty is practical work; for when the art of medicine is needed by the suffering and the dying it is no question of mere theoretical knowledge and extraneous acquirement. But skill in the commonest art is not to be attained without much practice, far less in the complicated and difficult art of healing, where every case presents some peculiarities. To practice it successfully, we must have made our home at our bedside, and, if I may say so, have lived with disease, observing it in all its forms and changes."

from *JAMA* (May 23/30), 2007;297:2200

Even though this quote is from the turn of the last century, Gull touches on several important points that remain active issues in medicine today. Many of these issues are the topics discussed in subsequent chapters in this book. For example, the struggle to balance science and art in life is the focus of Chapter 8, and the pursuit of a humanistic approach to end-of-life care is the focus of Chapter 14. For now, as a starting point in the discussion of the artistic side of medicine, let's take a moment and consider the importance of incorporating an artistic component in the doctor's bedside manner (which is probably the most pressing issue brought up by Gull in the above quote).

Bedside manner is a term that represents the complex human interaction encompassing many of the aspects of the caregiver–patient relationship including communication, body language, and other difficult-to-teach humanistic skill sets. Interestingly, less than optimal doctor–patient interactions have been shown to increase patient complaints and malpractice claims. A more detailed view of the doctor–patient relationship is explored in Chapter 10, but suffice it to say patients have long recognized that a physician's poor bedside manner can severely impact the treatment of disease. Despite this knowledge, it took more than 100 years after Gull's death before the United States formally recognized the importance of teaching medical students how to optimize their bedside manner as part of the medical school curriculum. In 2004, the United States Medical Licensing Exam began a mandatory clinical skills test, which grades students on their ability to effectively communicate and interact with patients. Interestingly, this test is actually performed on actors who feign disease, thereby further blurring the boundaries of medicine and the arts.

In summary, music is as much a science as medicine is an art. In this chapter, we have largely focused on the scientific basis of music; however, the remaining chapters in this book address the positive influence of integrating the arts into the field of medicine and, more specifically, caring for the cancer patient. Both caregivers and patients can benefit from achieving a balance of science and art in life, and music is one medium that can bring it all together.

CHAPTER 3

Music Therapy

Joanie M. Hope, MD and Nimesh P. Nagarsheth, MD

What comes to your mind when you think about the phrase *music and medicine*? Most people we have polled think about music therapy. This makes sense because, in this day and age, music therapy has developed into a free-standing field in the modern healthcare system. But how would you define music therapy? Where did it come from? And, what are the benefits? These are just some of the tough questions we explore in this chapter as we take you through a journey in this continuously evolving field.

The influence of music in the healthcare setting is not a new concept. In fact, there is evidence of humans exploring the healing powers of music dating back to ancient times. From a practical standpoint, in addition to describing the mathematical relationship of musical tones (discussed in Chapter 2), Pythagoras is also considered the father of music therapy. He and his followers (Pythagoreans) were considered experts in music, and were the first to suggest the combination of a healthy diet and music to achieve harmony of the body and soul. It was from this concept that music therapy was born.

Healthy Diet

In terms of a healthy diet, Pythagoras kept a diet that was high in fruits and strictly vegetarian. Over 2000 years later, scientific evidence has now demonstrated a diet high in fruits and low in meats decreases the risk of developing cancer. While this is not meant to imply that all meat products are unhealthy, clearly Pythagoras was ahead of his time in terms of understanding the role of eating habits on one's health and cancer risk, and adds credibility to his teachings.

In terms of the mysterious healing powers of music, Pythagoras said, "Rhythm subsists within the mind, and the mind exerts a powerful influence over the health of the body." This statement has been an inspiration for many artists and healers, and provides a direct explanation for how music can affect the physical healing process. Some of the more recent data demonstrating the role of music on this very real connection between mind and body healing are discussed below.

Although music therapy was practiced in some form 2,500 years ago, music therapy as a modern field of study has only been recently developed. Music was first introduced as a therapeutic modality during World War I to help treat soldiers with "shell shock," a mental condition now known as post-traumatic stress disorder. As described in the *New York Times* in 1918, doctors at Columbia University designed an experiment under "scientific auspices" that consisted of a concert by some of the top local talent for soldiers whose nerves had been shattered by the stresses of trench life. The effect of this musical intervention was encouraging: "Some of the most hopeless cases were brightened and cheered" and people were noted to be "humming snatches of the songs or whistling bits of tunes they heard that day."

During World War II, a more institutionalized approach to music therapy was incorporated by veteran's hospitals with a systematic exposure of patients to music in an effort to boost morale and enhance psychological well-being. Indeed, the academic world took notice, and the first formalized music therapy curriculum was established in 1944 at Michigan State University followed by the first professional association in 1950. Today, there are close to 4,000 practicing music therapists and over 70 degree-granting programs approved by the American Music Therapy Association.

As doctors, we are trained to perpetually ask ourselves: Do our actions actually help our patients? Or in this case, does music really heal? And if so, can we prove this in a scientific fashion? When

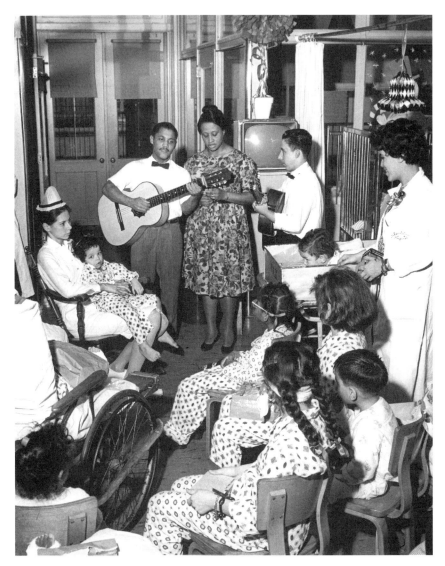

Figure 3-1. Musicians entertain patients on the pediatric ward at Mount Sinai Hospital in the 1960s.
Courtesy of the Mount Sinai Archives, New York, NY.

performing a search for the key term *music therapy* on PubMed—the most commonly used academic database used by doctors—2,740 hits were generated as of this writing. A search for the key terms *music and cancer* yielded 270 academic papers. Within this body of work is scientific data suggesting that music triggers physiologic

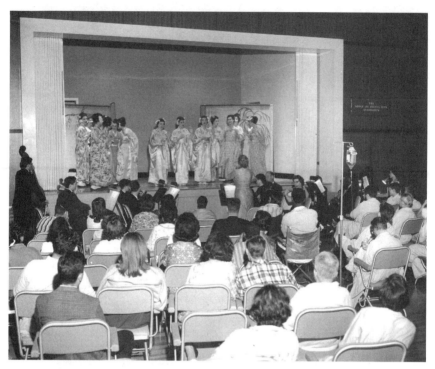

Figure 3-2. Musical and theatrical productions entered the hospital setting in the mid-1900s to entertain patients and their loved ones.
Courtesy of the Mount Sinai Archives, New York, NY.

responses that: 1) reduce blood pressure, heart rate, and pace of breathing; 2) occupy the neurotransmitters that are used to transmit pain messages to the brain and thereby decrease the perception of pain; 3) diminish levels of stress, fear, and anxiety; and 4) increase feelings of self-worth and ease symptoms of depression. For cancer patients in particular, music therapy has been shown to reduce chemotherapy-induced nausea and vomiting, enhance relaxation, diminish pain, and help patients and their families adjust to life with cancer.

A comprehensive review of 51 well-conducted studies evaluating whether music aids in pain relief concluded that listening to music reduces both pain intensity and narcotic (pain medicine) requirements in patients. In the music therapy world, participating in the creation of music may be just as important as listening to music, and both are emphasized in patients who are physically and emotionally able. In fact, in a recent study of children with cancer, an active musical engagement strategy was more beneficial than passively listening to music or audio storybooks.

Because music can have such positive effects for patients, one might also wonder if it could help the stress levels, coping abilities, and performance of healthcare providers? In other words, could music help doctors be better doctors? Music has interwoven with modern medicine in many different forms. In 1914, music made its first entrance into the operating room. But with regard to music during surgery, the jury is still out. In one survey of 171 doctors and nurses, 63% regularly listened to music in the operating room with over 50% selecting classical music. Older doctors preferred quieter music, and almost 80% of respondents believed that music made the operating room calmer and more efficient. On the other hand, a well-respected trial exposing junior surgeons to music while learning minimally invasive surgery techniques concluded that music had a distracting effect on novice surgeons and should be prohibited during teaching procedures. On a personal note, we believe in the beneficial role of music in the operating room and believe that the rhythm of music adds to the chemistry of the surgery and results in the best overall outcomes for our patients.

When patients have input in the song selection and are not receiving general anesthesia, music has been shown to decrease the need for pain medication during and after surgery. And with the help of music therapy, some minor surgeries are successfully being performed at select institutions without any anesthesia at all. Music in the operating room was brought into vogue in 1997 when President Bill Clinton underwent knee surgery to repair a traumatic tendon injury at the National Naval Medical Center in Bethesda, Maryland. During his 2-hour procedure, President Clinton and his doctors listened to the country music of Lyle Lovett. His doctors even reported that Clinton was requesting specific songs throughout the surgery. Although often overlooked on the many Internet blogs commenting on his experience, President Clinton did benefit from the use of regional anesthesia (an epidural) during this procedure and did not rely solely on music for pain control. Nonetheless, President Clinton was described as feeling well and being in a pleasant mood following his surgery, and this was largely attributed to him enjoying music during his surgery.

Many other well-known and respected individuals have helped bring music and medicine into the mainstream public eye. Dr. Oliver Sacks, a professor of neurology at Columbia University, brought international attention to the positive relationship between music and medicine through his publications regarding patients suffering from Parkinson's disease. These patients experience disorders of timing in which their movements can be too fast, too slow, or completely frozen. Dr. Sacks demonstrated that exposure to the regular tempo and rhythm of music can help them momentarily restore normal motion. Similarly, people with Tourette's syndrome are prone to sudden and uncontrolled verbal and physical outbursts, and can become controlled and tic-free while listening to (or performing) music. These amazing results echo the words of 19th-century German philosopher, Friedrich Wilhelm Nietzche, who said, "We listen to music with our muscles." While this is undoubtedly true, we also listen to music with our hearts. Music is profoundly emotionally evocative, and as such, can have an impressive impact on people with Alzheimer's disease, autism, and frontal lobe disorders. On the flip side, music also can be over-stimulating and lead to seizures and hallucinations in rare cases. Just as with most good things in life, even music is not perfect.

As music is one of the oldest forms of communication, it comes as no surprise that leading experts in the field of oncology use music as a medium to help patients understand medical concepts. For example, when asked to describe what distinguishes a cancer cell from a normal cell in the human body, Dr. Larry Norton, Deputy Physician and Chief at Memorial Sloan-Kettering Cancer Center, states that cancer cells are only slightly different than normal cells and provides his patients with an analogy of listening to 40 players in an orchestra. By simply changing the notes from just one violinist, the entire orchestra sounds terrible. And that, says Dr. Norton, is an excellent parallel of how the genetic make up of a cancer cell is different from a normal cell. In general, cancer cells possess very small alterations that unfortunately lead to drastic changes in the way cells behave. Importantly, we have found that simple musical-based analogies like this one go a long way in helping patients understand the disease process and the challenges we face as clinicians and researchers in the fight against cancer.

Overall, we believe wholeheartedly in the concepts of using music as a medium to help cancer patients heal, and to help doctors be better doctors. In line with this thought process, N.E.D. recorded our first studio album in 2009. A track from this album, "Rhythm Heals" (see lyrics below), is our modern day commentary on the eternal role of music in the fight against cancer.

Rhythm Heals (original version)
© 2009 by N.E.D.
Lyrics by Joanie M. Hope
Music by Joanie M. Hope and Nimesh P. Nagarsheth

(*verse 1*)
Dreams of youth . . . Resurrected
The length of travel . . . Unexpected
The hierarchy . . . Disrespected
Truth be told . . . Rhythm heals!

(*chorus*)
Rhythm heals
Rhythm heals
Rhythm heals
Rhythm heals
Rhythm heals
Rhythm heals

The outcome is . . . Anticipated
Just for now . . . Lets be elated
The benefit . . . Always debated
Truth be told . . . Rhythm heals!

(*chorus*)
Rhythm heals
Rhythm heals
Rhythm heals
Rhythm heals
Rhythm heals
Rhythm heals

I don't know you . . . Do you know me?
Come together . . . Music and disease
It's enough . . . To fill the need
Truth be told . . . Rhythm heals!

(*Bridge*)
Piled six high in that last cab to survive
On that hot sweet July after jamming all night
The skeleton streets still echoed our beats
We were trashed to the bone from our rock and roll moans
We were free!

(*chorus*)
We were free
We were free
We were free
Rhythm heals
Rhythm heals
Rhythm heals

These lyrics were written in the summer of 2008 shortly after our band played a gig for our colleagues at a cancer meeting on the Magnificent Mile in Chicago. The song captures the incredible chemistry and feeling of elation we experienced channeling through our bodies as we merged our dual passions: fighting cancer and playing music.

The first verse opens with expressions of our feelings of having the rare second chance at the childhood dream of playing music professionally. With six busy cancer surgeons spread across the United States, even a simple rehearsal required months of planning ("length of travel . . . unexpected"). But for us, we knew deep down the effort was worth it as our music has always been from the heart and soul ("Truth be told"). From that pure and honest energy, we ignited the passion that would get us through the many obstacles we faced (geographic, financial, etc.), and through the many doubts thrown our way as to whether or not this project would be successful ("The benefit . . . always debated"). The final verse of "Rhythm Heals" illustrates our realization of the successful integration of music and medicine to help patients, and is an invitation to all those listening to join our fight ("Come together . . . music and disease").

On a personal note, a memorable story of the band is told in the bridge of the song, which describes our experience after rehearsing for over 12 hours in the outskirts of Chicago only to find out that no cabs were available to take us back to our hotel. When we finally flagged down a taxi, all six of us piled in with instruments in hand, making for a magical and unforgettable night. The lyrics to this song are our message to you: Rhythm Heals.

CHAPTER 4

Jazz Improvisation: An Example of Music and Medicine Working Together in Harmony

Nimesh P. Nagarsheth, MD

You may be wondering why jazz is the only field of music that has its own dedicated chapter in this book. I would be wondering the same thing if I were you. After all, by now you can guess that my favorite type of music is rock, so why not a chapter saluting 'for those about to rock'? Of course, to the fans each genre of music, whether it be classical, folk, rap, hip-hop, country, techno, heavy metal, or other, is special in its own way. But what makes jazz unique is that it is the only form of music that truly permeates into all of the different genres of modern music. In this sense, you can almost think of jazz as the all-encompassing genre. This is because jazz is all about freedom, and in jazz, anything goes.

Jazz was born around the early 1900s in New Orleans, Louisiana. Why New Orleans of all places? New Orleans had all of the elements in place to ignite the spark of something creative and new. It began as a cultural phenomenon originating from the integration of two very different African-American socioeconomic classes: the poorly educated and financially disadvantaged African Americans who had been recently emancipated lived west of Canal Street and had little if any formal training in music. In contrast, the highly educated and financially well-to-do Creoles (European-educated African Americans) lived east of Canal Street and had extensive formal training in music. Due to political, cultural, and racially-charged events that had been taking place in the United States during that time, New Orleans passed a segregation law, forcing those two cultures to live together west of this city's divide. As a result, European and African musical influences soon became integrated, and jazz was born.

Taking elements from the blues, ragtime, waltz, polka, opera, Spanish flare, gospel, and the lower class' working songs, jazz brought forward the concepts of swing and improvisation into modern music. As a reflection of the times, shortly after its birth in New Orleans jazz emerged in several other cities across the United States including Chicago, St. Louis, Kansas City, and of course New York City. Over the next several decades, the various forms of jazz we now enjoy today took shape and include styles such as Dixieland, swing (big band), bebop, progressive, Latin, rock, and free jazz. The importance of jazz as an art form is now well-established and, in 1987, the U.S. Congress passed a resolution recognizing jazz as a "national American treasure" that deserves attention and support to assure its preservation.

As you can see, the history of jazz is deeply rooted in the history of the United States, and this story is an ideal example of how music reflects life. Jazz emerged as a musical response to a troubled society struggling with important issues, and is the product of democracy, freedom of expression, integration of cultures, and the free exchange of ideas. Today, jazz crosses all divides (both real and imagined) including those related to geography, race, culture, education, and socioeconomic status. In addition, jazz serves as a powerful political and humanitarian tool. In fact, jazz is at the center of one of the greatest humanitarian success stories of modern times, uniting music and medicine to help fight disease. If you've never heard this before, you are not alone. In fact, even though I studied medicine and jazz separately for most of my adult life, I was not aware of the incredible working relationship between jazz and medicine until I finished my medical training. Then one day, **out of nowhere**, I suddenly found myself on the frontlines of the jazz healthcare crisis, and became a part of incredibly inspiring story.

> Some of the greatest opportunities in life can appear from this nebulous place we often refer to as "out of nowhere." Whether you call it fate, destiny, chance, coincidence, being in the right place at the right time, or just plain luck, sometimes it's better not to question why things occur, but rather just make like a drum and roll with it.

When I first signed on as an attending physician in gynecologic oncology at the Mount Sinai Medical Center in New York, I was unaware of the opportunities hidden in the woodwork of my new position that would eventually lead me to the very heart and soul of jazz. However, in addition to taking on new responsibilities including teaching (students, residents, and fellows), performing research, and treating patients, I knew early on that this position might require me to staff (provide clinical services for) a nearby satellite hospital away from the main campus, and I was excited about this opportunity.

An Interesting Fact

Because there are only a limited number of gynecologic oncologists in the United States, patients traditionally had to commute (sometimes long distances) to centrally located, major medical centers to receive their care. However, in an effort to improve the quality of life of patients by increasing accessibility, gynecologic oncologists throughout the country have made a paradigm shift in the way they deliver care, and many now provide the same intense surgical and medical care that had usually been reserved for the major academic centers in smaller community hospitals.

The powers that be quickly assigned me to staff Englewood Hospital and Medical Center. Although located only 20 minutes from Manhattan (just across the George Washington Bridge) in northern New Jersey, I had never visited the city of Englewood. So, in an effort to familiarize myself with the community, one Friday afternoon I jumped in my car and scouted out the location of the hospital and the surrounding area. On my way home, I passed by Bennett

Studios, located just near the train tracks passing through downtown Englewood. Although I had heard of Bennett Studios, it wasn't until this very moment that I realized this incredible facility was situated just down the street from the site of my new surgical practice. Unable to resist the urge, I pulled over and walked inside to take a look. One the members of the studio staff greeted me at the front entrance and offered a short tour. He explained to me that Tony Bennett's son ran the studio, and occasionally Tony Bennett himself would make an appearance. He went on to tell me how some of the outstanding musicians of our time have spent long hours in this very building recording some very well-known songs and albums. When he learned I was in town preparing to start a gynecologic oncology practice at Englewood Hospital, his face lit up with a smile and he told me how in this community, music and medicine have pulled together like never before, generating amazing stories of hope and altruism. And with that statement he welcomed me to Englewood, the sacred healing ground for jazz musicians around the world.

What was he talking about? Through my new position at Englewood Hospital and Medical Center, I had stumbled onto one of the greatest success stories of the integration of music and medicine, and jazz encompassed it all. In time, I would become familiar with the incredible history that made Englewood the place where jazz heals. Was it fate that I had been assigned to Englewood Hospital? Like I said, sometimes it's better not to ask why. I just made like a drum and rolled with it.

The Jazz Foundation of America (www.jazzfoundation.org) began in 1989, when five individuals came together to create an organization dedicated to the preservation of the art of jazz. The foundation quickly discovered that one of the most urgent issues facing jazz musicians across the United States was financial instability. These musicians were not in music for the money but rather for the love of jazz. They would often perform night after night at local clubs collecting only tips or minimal reimbursements. This setup prevented them from having formal pension or retirement plans, and many were unable to afford basic health insurance. Even some of the well-known jazz greats with big-time hits never realized the financial rewards they deserved as many had signed away the rights for their songs. Instead of collecting royalties, these jazz artists had agreed to receive a one-time payment for their recording session. They were true artists in every sense of the word, playing for the love of music and "singing for the love of singing."

In the 1990s, the reality of the jazz healthcare crisis came to a breaking point. With many legendary jazz musicians hitting retirement age and requiring significant medical attention, a major public health issue ensued and took center stage in the music community. Flooding the healthcare system and delving further into debt, these jazz musicians needed help fast. Fundraising efforts began in 1992 and the Jazz Foundation of America activated the Jazz Musicians' Emergency Fund. But, like cancer outgrowing its blood supply, the need for help was growing far greater than the resources that were available at that time. The jazz community needed a miracle to reverse this mounting problem. That miracle came in 1993 at Englewood Hospital and Medical Center through the magical workings of an incredible doctor-patient relationship involving a trumpet player named Dizzy, and his medical oncologist Dr. Frank Forte.

Dizzy Gillespie was not just any trumpet player—he was a world-class musician. Although most well-known for his bent (forty-five degree bell) trumpet, Dizzy was a bandleader, composer, and a major contributor to the development of bebop and jazz. In February 1992, at the age of 74, Dizzy Gillespie's health began to rapidly decline, and he suffered from symptoms including nausea, vomiting, and weakness. One month later, he was diagnosed with pancreatic cancer at Englewood Hospital. After his surgery, Dizzy began an intensive treatment regimen with chemotherapy and supportive care under the supervision of Dr. Frank Forte. What made this doctor-patient combination unique was that both the patient and the doctor were musical legends in their own right. In addition to being an outstanding physician, Dr. Forte is an accomplished guitarist and renowned jazz musician. Using both his music and medical expertise, Dr. Forte was able to foster the creative jazz environment from which great solos (or in this case, creative thoughts and ideas) are born.

Just before undergoing another surgery for his worsening disease in September 1992, Dizzy had a creative thought that later would become his legacy. Recognizing the need to help his fellow musicians who were not as fortunate as him, he asked Dr. Forte to help him figure out a way to provide free medical care to the indigent jazz musicians of the world. Dizzy wanted to help in any way possible, and while he didn't have enough money to tackle this massive project on his own, he was able to contribute something far more valuable: his name. Unfortunately, in January 1993, Dizzy Gillespie died of pancreatic cancer, but he never lost sight of what was important in life, and his legacy will live on forever. In his last few days in the hospital, when reflecting on his life, Dizzy told his good friend's daughter, "It's been a great gig."

Shortly after Dizzy's request to help his colleagues in need, Dr. Forte and the Englewood Hospital set up the Dizzy Gillespie Memorial Fund. With close to 50 doctors volunteering their services "in the spirit of Dizzy Gillespie" along with the hospital supplying the necessary medical support and backing, this program has been an overwhelming success. To date, the program has provided care to over 1,000 musicians and has donated over five million dollars in free medical care to the jazz artists from around the world. Working closely with the Jazz Foundation of America, Englewood Hospital and the Dizzy Gillespie program continues to receive a steady flow of patient referrals and financial support, and both patients and hospital staff benefit from regular jazz performances from some of the greatest jazz performers of our time.

Moving forward in the spirit of Dizzy Gillespie, in 2007 a new music project entitled "Jazz Therapy" was started by Motéma Music, a record company based out of New York City. This series features recorded tracks (and live performances) from prominent jazz musicians and serves as an ongoing source of fundraising for the Dizzy Gillespie Memorial Fund. Volume 1 of Jazz Therapy was released in 2008 and is entitled "Smile." This work features the master guitarists Gene Bertoncini and Roni Ben-Hur (available at www.motema.com). In the CD insert of this album, an inspiring quote from Doctor Frank Forte sums up this model relationship between music and medicine at Englewood Hospital.

"Medicine is more than tests, diagnoses, and drugs. It has been all about healing since the beginning. Healing implies concern, love, trust, and the powers to encourage the infirm to rise to getting better, to restore the wholeness of self again. The relationship of our hospital with the Jazz Foundation of America has brought these positive experiences in healing and is magical. Working with the performers and all the generous people who put this together proves that it's about doing good for others and making sick people better. Heaven knows that music is a force that brings renewal to the sick and also to the staff who treat them. The music spurs on the caregivers and family members too. We know this for sure at Englewood Hospital."

The Jazz Foundation of America and Englewood Hospital relationship is just one of many instances where music and medicine have been successfully integrated for the purposes of improving the quality of life of patients, and advancing medical research and clinical care. In the spirit of jazz ("anything goes"), I would like to share with you two other inspiring stories that have led to the creation of foundations that are harnessing the power of music to benefit medicine. In each of these organizations, music has served to unite people behind an important cause. As with most Cinderella stories, these organizations started with passion and have blossomed through the hard work and dedication of their many supporters.

The first inspiring story comes from Tony Martell, a music industry executive, who describes in his own words the creation of the T.J. Martell Foundation as a result of his struggle dealing with the loss of his son and his determination to make a difference in the fight against cancer.

Dear Friends,

When my son, T.J., passed away in 1975 at the age of 19 due to leukemia, my life felt displaced and the pain unbearable. It was only the promise I had made to him that kept me afloat amidst such a devastating personal tragedy and filled me with purpose—to raise one million dollars for lifesaving cancer research.

T.J. wanted to fortify and expand the critical research that had enabled him to survive 2 years beyond his original prognosis. He understood so well the significance of his terrible disease and its impact on not only himself, but on the lives of so many other young victims and their families.

With the help of artists and friends within and outside the music industry, several fundraising events were organized and eventually, the T.J. Martell Foundation was founded. Since its formation, we have raised nearly a quarter of a billion dollars in support of innovative cancer research at eight extraordinary research laboratories throughout the country. Groundbreaking progress is being made every day, and I now see that a real cure is becoming much less of an impossible journey.

It has been many years since the one million dollar mark was achieved—but for my beloved son T.J., and for everyone else who has undergone the experience of cancer, leukemia, or AIDS, I pledge that the T.J. Martell Foundation will not rest until a true cure is discovered.

Tony Martell
Founder, T.J. Martell Foundation
www.tjmartellfoundation.org

Today, the T.J. Martell Foundation is an incredibly successful, internationally recognized, non-profit collaborative organization dedicated to funding research and improving the quality of life of people with cancer and AIDS. Originating from a fundraising event at Buddy Rich's club in New York City in 1975, the foundation has emerged as one of the world's leading sponsors of innovative research using funding and publicity generated from famous musical talents and celebrities. Similar to the creative environment from which the art form of jazz emerged, the foundation has created a forum where scientists from around the world can meet and freely exchange ideas at regular intervals to push the boundaries of medicine and science. Researchers receiving funding from the T.J. Martell Foundation are encouraged to explore options that may be considered outside the box and have enjoyed incredible success in this creative environment. As a token of his incredible commitment in the fight against cancer and AIDS, the Mount Sinai School of Medicine granted Tony Martell an honorary humanitarian degree in 2009.

In a similar fashion, another inspiring story comes from Ken Trush, the co-founder of Daniel's Music Foundation. Ken describes in his own words the ordeal he went through watching his son fight a serious medical illness, and shares how this experience inspired the creation of Daniel's Music Foundation.

Dear Friends,

Music has always been a big part of my life. But as with the majority of people, music became more of a passive activity as I grew older. Sure, I played the recorder, guitar, and tuba while I was in elementary and junior high school, but as soon as adolescence kicked in my musical experience became limited to listening to other people's songs and creations. Little did I know, however, that on March 9, 1997, this would be the start of a great change in how I interacted with music.

It was a Sunday afternoon, and spring was in the air. My oldest son, Daniel, who was 12 at that time, was playing basketball at his school's gym. My wife, Nancy, and my younger son, Michael, were also in attendance. About 20 minutes into the game, Daniel took a shot and came running off the court holding his head. I thought he was upset about missing the shot, but instead subsequently found out that one of his five brain aneurysms had exploded. Daniel was as close to death's door as one could get. In fact, on the second night, the doctor woke me up at the hospital and told me to get my family to say goodbye. The pressure in his head was so high that effectively he had no blood or oxygen going to his brain. Daniel survived that night and remained in a coma for 30 days. During the darkest hours, as I was serenaded by a symphony of beeps and buzzers, I turned to music to comfort my soul. I would watch Daniel, and play music for both he and I. I found the Gloria Estefan CD "Destiny" to be particularly soothing and relaxing and would play it sometimes three or four times a day. A few weeks into Daniel's coma, I lost the CD and received another copy 3 months later for my birthday. When I played it again, Daniel now awake, knew many of the words to the songs. Apparently, the music had somehow been able to penetrate his brain even when he was in a coma.

As Daniel continued to progress in his rehabilitation—he was in the hospital for almost 1 year—music became even more important to us. Music became the vehicle for us to communicate and for Daniel to express himself, to gain self-esteem, and build confidence. It also allowed him to be creative and innovative, as he learned a new instrument, the keyboard. Music also helped Daniel with his memory, as he was able to remember songs, melodies, and music theory much better than both the written and spoken word. As time went on, an inspiration came to both of us that led our family to start a non-profit music foundation, aptly named Daniel's Music Foundation. The organization provides free music instruction classes for people with disabilities in the NYC area. We have seen first hand how music can enhance people's lives and now, 12 years after his injury, Daniel has dedicated his life to helping others through music. As for me, after 40 years of being a "passive music listener," I am also learning to play a new instrument, the keyboard. I am enjoying playing more than ever. And who is my instructor? Daniel, of course!

Ken Trush
Co-Founder
Daniel's Music Foundation
www.danielsmusic.org

Daniel's Music Foundation is a non-profit organization whose mission is to provide people with medical disabilities a comfortable, educational, and social environment where members can enjoy, learn, and practice the joys of music together. In 2006, the organization started out with one keyboard class and a dream to help others through music. The demand and membership has quickly grown and now this group offers 18 music instruction classes for its members and provides a variety of other services.

Jazz teaches us that great things can come from creativity and freedom of expression. It is this spirit that Daniel's Music Foundation tries to harness, and it is the same spirit from which the T.J. Martell Foundation was created. Jazz links all styles of music and is the canvas from which great ideas are born. Whether a musician or a patient, you should always hold onto your creativity and your sense of self. After all, that is your jazz solo in the song of life!

PART II

The Music Lessons— Getting Started

Coping with the Initial Diagnosis of Cancer: The Song Writing Workshop Approach to the Grieving Process

Nimesh P. Nagarsheth, MD

In her 1969 book entitled, *On Death and Dying*, Elisabeth Kubler-Ross introduced the concept of the five stages of grief. Adapted from a previous four-stage description by Bowlby and Parkes several years prior, the Kubler-Ross five-stage model is denial, anger, bargaining, depression, and acceptance (see Table 5-1). A more recent four-stage theory of grief that appears on the National Cancer Institute's Web site describes adaptations by Jacobs and includes the categories of shock and numbness, yearning and searching, disorganization and despair, and reorganization. Although several grief theories have been proposed, the Kubler-Ross model remains very familiar to the general public.

Importantly, these stages of grief can be applied to virtually any life stressor or tragedy. In addition to those dealing with death and illness, patients with any form of significant trauma or personal loss, including job loss, divorce, and other life-changing events, may go through one or more of these five stages.

Table 5-1 Three Models of Grief, Loss, and Bereavement

Model	Stage	Thoughts and Feelings
Kubler-Ross Five Stages of Grief	1. Denial	This isn't happening.
	2. Anger	Why is this happening to me?
	3. Bargaining	I promise I'll be a better person *if* . . .
	4. Depression	I am sad.
	5. Acceptance	*I'm ready* for whatever comes, and am ready to move forward with my life.
Bowlby and Parkes Four Stages of Grief	1. Shock and Numbness	Anesthetic affect, withdrawal, depersonalization, unreality.
	2. Yearning and Searching	Fruitless pining for whom is lost and then intellectually realizing the person has passed.
	3. Disorganization and Despair	Enduring, waxing, and waning feelings of mourning and severe pain of loss.
	4. Reorganization	Incorporation of the loss, recognition that life goes on; redefining one's life without the person.
National Cancer Institute Process of Bereavement (Jacobs modification with emphasis on separation anxiety)	1. Shock and Numbness	Difficulty believing that the death has occurred; feeling stunned and numb.
	2. Yearning and Searching	Separation anxiety; ongoing frustration disappointment at the impossibility of bringing back the deceased.
	3. Disorganization and Despair	Feelings of depression and difficulty moving on. Difficulty in staying focused.
	4. Reorganization	Finding new paradigms of living at peace without the deceased.

Sources: Adapted from
1. Kubler-Ross E. *On Death and Dying*. New York: Scribner; 1969.
2. Kirkley-Best E. *Grief, Bereavement & Loss*. © 2004 Elizabeth Kirkley-Best. Available at http://www.forgottengrief.com/griefoverview.html. Accessed May 9, 2009.
3. National Cancer Institute. *Loss, Grief, and Bereavement (PDQ®)*. Available at http://www.cancer.gov/cancertopics/pdq/supportivecare/bereavement/Patient/page6. Accessed May 9, 2009.

Receiving news of the diagnosis of cancer is probably one of the most stressful events you will ever experience in your life, and will likely bring you into some form of the grieving process. Taking the time to understand the grieving process will help you navigate through the natural course of events that you can expect to feel as you deal with the diagnosis, treatment, and long-term implications related to your illness. An artistic approach to exploring these stages of grief is an effective way to grasp the complex nature of this phenomenon and begin your healing process.

Although presented in order here, Kubler-Ross acknowledged that patients may not experience the stages of grief in order, and that not every patient may experience every stage. Generally, however, patients going through the grieving process usually pass through at least two of these stages.

Using music as a tool to help patients manage the grieving process is not a new concept, and scientific studies have shown that patients can benefit from this approach. In 2006, Dalton and Krout published their work on the development and implementation of the Grief Song-Writing Process (GSWP). This study focused on bereaved adolescents and was divided into three parts. First, the themes and core concerns that emerged in over 100 songs that had been written by adolescents undergoing individual music therapy sessions were analyzed. The authors then compared these themes with existing grieving models (such as those outlined above) and created a new integrated grieving model (derived partly from this musical approach) that included the stages of understanding, feeling, remembering, integrating, and growing. Finally, based on the information above, the researchers created and implemented a seven-session song writing workshop. The adolescents were asked to write original lyrics and songs based on each of the five stages of grieving that had been identified through the musical inspiration, and greatly benefited from this exercise. Although this study focused on bereaved adolescents, there is no reason to believe that cancer patients going through the grieving process would not benefit from similar exercises of writing songs.

Channeling your emotional energy (whether positive or negative) into a song can be extremely therapeutic for the mind and body. Even if you are not musically inclined, simply putting your thoughts down in writing (lyrics) can be a productive and constructive way to express your thoughts and concerns while going through the fight against cancer. An easy way to begin this therapeutic process is to simply keep a journal of your experiences.

Following our own advice, we as cancer doctors decided to channel our emotions and thoughts into song. Similar to the GSWP model as outlined on page 42, our band of gynecologic oncologists (N.E.D.) wrote a song called "Third Person Reality" that outlines the complexities of breaking bad news to patients (specifically communicating the initial diagnosis of cancer). Interestingly, my original version of lyrics from this song elicited strong emotions and opinions from every band member in our group as well as our producer and the president of our record company. During our first rehearsal, the lyrics and musical construction of this song was the most debated and contested out of any song that is on our debut album. While this may not surprise you, given the emotional nature of this song, let's take a moment to analyze the original lyrical content to better understand what you (and your physician) may feel while struggling with the initial diagnosis of cancer.

> *Third Person Reality* (original version)
> © 2009 by N.E.D.
> Lyrics by Nimesh P. Nagarsheth
> Music by Nimesh P. Nagarsheth and Joanie M. Hope
>
> (*Verse 1*)
> It starts with denial
> There must be some mistake
> Check the lab, check the name
> Double check the date

I read just the opposite
On the net the other day
Down the street
That doc over there
What does he have to say?

(*Verse 2*)
Anger sets in
Whose fault can this be?
Beer, wine, and gin
The struggle to be free

Legal terms begin
Tensions run high
Fear of the end
Look towards the sky

(*Chorus*)
Close the door
It's time to shatter another dream
If these 4 walls could talk
You would know what I mean

This is where lives change
This is where we became
A Third Person Reality

(*Verse 3*)
Let's bargain a while
As the clouds settle in
How much for a day?
A week, a month or a year?

Nothing's for sale
In this store we're in
Where life is as precious
As family and friends

(*Verse 4*)
And now you look so sad
You try to think happy thoughts
You're no longer mad
Ready to fight, but have not fought

There are ways to cope with the sadness
Medicine, support and such
The rays of hope and the madness
Feel the power of the healing touch

(*Chorus*)
Close the door
It's time to shatter another dream
If these 4 walls could talk
You would know what I mean

This is where lives change
This is where we became
A Third Person Reality

(*Bridge*)
He, she, they or them
Just keep it far from me
He, she, they or them
Third Person Reality

(*Verse 5*)
The final resolution
Acceptance is the key
Draw from those around you
Take what you need from me

Measure success one day at a time
And together we'll get to a better place
Put your hand in mine
Put your hand in mine

(*Chorus*)
Close the door
It's time to shatter another dream
If these 4 walls could talk
You would know what I mean

This is where lives change
This is where we became
A Third Person Reality

"Third Person Reality" was originally written as five verses, three choruses, and one bridge. Each verse represents one stage of the grieving process as described by Kubler-Ross (see Table 5-1). As you read through the verses, hopefully you will gain a better understanding of some of the common themes we have seen from cancer patients. For example, after initially learning of their cancer diagnosis, patients often question the correctness of their diagnosis ("There must be some mistake") or wish to seek a second opinion ("Down the street, that doc over there, What does he have to say?"). This is the denial stage, and it usually passes quickly. Denial is often followed by feelings of anger, and a desire to place blame on someone or something else for developing cancer. Patients frequently ask whether their primary care doctor missed the diagnosis, or whether this cancer should have been found sooner. In the vast majority of cases, no wrong doing was ever committed by the referring physician, and fortunately patients rarely pursue legal action in cases where it is not indicated. Nonetheless, anger is probably the most difficult stage of grief to watch a patient experience, and if not recognized or handled carefully by the doctor, this stage can result in long-term damage of the doctor-patient relationship.

The bargaining stage of grief can present in many different forms, but often it is often expressed through monetary value. For example, patients will sometimes ask (and be willing to pay out-of-pocket) for extra and unnecessary tests. Ironically, deviating from the standard of care may actually result in treatment delays and worse outcomes if pursued. On a personal note, I find the most disturbing part of this song to be the suggestion that some patients believe that money can buy time. ("How much for a day? A week, a month or a year?") Fortunately, healthcare reform in the United States is now taking center stage in terms of making excellent care available to anyone who needs it.

Patients receiving the diagnosis of cancer may enter a state of depression. Fortunately, this stage is usually short-lived and rarely results in serious consequences. Most patients are often able to recover from their depression with the support of family and friends, as well as with the occasional antidepressant medication therapy.

> If you feel you may be in a state of serious depression, please contact your physician immediately.

Finally, acceptance represents the ultimate goal of successfully going through the grieving process. Patients who reach acceptance early on are able to resume a productive and active lifestyle, and for most patients measuring success "one day at a time" are words to live by.

In the chorus of "Third Person Reality," the doctor voices the frustration and despair of dealing with the repeated task of telling patients they have cancer. In a detached and almost perfunctory manner, the doctor tells his assistant to "close the door, it's time to shatter another dream." The doctor is unable to deal with the intensity of facing the patient directly when delivering this bad news, and emotionally detaches himself from the situation by viewing himself as an onlooker (a third person in the room). While physically he remains seated in front of the patient, his mind spiritually leaves his body in a manner similar to that depicted in movies when a person's soul leaves his body in a ghost-like fashion.

Although this defense mechanism provides a quick fix for the doctor in terms of not having to internalize the patient's struggle, this process also prevents the doctor from making that personal connection which is so crucial for the healing touch. Fortunately, in the last verse of the song, the patient has reached a place of acceptance and the doctor has also gained a better understanding of the healing process. Together the patient and doctor finally make that necessary connection ("put your hand in mine"), which is needed to humanize the doctor-patient relationship and achieve the best outcome.

An important point that this song brings to light is that in addition to being catastrophic for you as a patient, conveying bad news may have severe consequences for your physician as well. This is because the art of delivering bad news is an interactive process between the doctor and patient, and the empathetic physician will often share the sense of struggle and pain that the patient experiences when grappling with the diagnosis. Although sharing in the patient's emotions can be a healthy process when performed carefully, the overly empathetic cancer doctor who delivers bad news on a daily basis can be overrun by the strong emotions this process elicits. It is common to encounter cancer doctors who have developed a hardened shell to protect themselves from the difficult social interactions they must face every day as a part of their job. Unfortunately, as depicted in "Third Person Reality," the defense mechanisms that some doctors develop in response to emotionally painful situations will prevent them from providing effective and compassionate care. Whether or not having a background in the arts has a positive impact on the doctor's ability to communicate effectively in times such as these remains to be determined, but physicians with an artistic background may have an advantage in this setting.

> Interestingly, over the past several years, medical schools around the country have developed programs designed to recruit students who show promise for becoming compassionate and humanistic physicians. These programs encourage prospective students to pursue undergraduate degrees in the humanities, social sciences, and the arts. In fact, the Humanities and Medicine Program at the Mount Sinai School of Medicine in New York is one of the most well-known programs of this kind. True to its name, students accepted into this program are guaranteed admission to medical school early in their undergraduate schooling, thereby allowing them to pursue a degree in the arts instead of pursuing the standard pre-med or science degree.

When the grieving process is not handled correctly, it can result in severe consequences. As such, I strongly encourage my patients to openly discuss their thoughts and feelings about how they are coping with the initial diagnosis of cancer and the other stressors in their life. Help is available for those who desire it, and grief counseling and/or grief therapy may be a good place to start. The National Cancer Institute (NCI) web site (www.cancer.gov) can be a valuable resource to learn more about these important treatment strategies. The goals and benefits of grief counseling and grief therapy are discussed below.

Grief counseling is designed to help patients work through the stages of grief by participating in individual or group counseling sessions. The major goals of grief counseling (as adapted from the NCI web site) are summarized below.

- Helping the patient to accept the event (i.e., cancer diagnosis) by helping him or her to talk about the event.
- Helping the patient to identify and express feelings related to the event (including anger, guilt, anxiety, helplessness, and sadness).
- Helping the patient to live with the event and to continue making decisions and function in daily life.
- Identifying and providing support at times that may be particularly stressful for the patient such as holidays, birthdays, and anniversaries.
- Educating the patient about the normal grieving process.
- Helping the patient to understand his or her methods of coping.
- Identifying coping problems the patient may experience and making recommendations for professional grief therapy if needed.

Grief therapy can be thought of as a more intensive form of grief counseling and is typically reserved for patients with severe grief reactions, and patients experiencing more significant difficulty coping with the inciting event. Similar to grief counseling, grief therapy can be performed through individual and/or group therapy sessions. Six basic methods utilized in grief therapy (as adapted from the NCI web site) are summarized below

- Helping the patient experience, express, and adjust to painful grief-related changes.
- Finding effective ways to cope with painful changes.
- Establishing a continuing relationship with the event (acceptance).
- Staying healthy, mentally and physically, and maintaining daily life activities.
- Re-establishing relationships and understanding that others may have difficulty understanding the situation.
- Developing a healthy image of oneself and the world around them.

In conclusion, receiving a diagnosis of cancer can be a traumatic experience for anyone, no matter how well-adjusted, successful, or grounded. Therefore, in coping with this major life stressor, it is only natural that you may experience one or more components of the stages of grief. However, by gaining a better understanding of the process through an artistic approach, you will be able to reach a place of acceptance faster, and remain in a better mental and physical health overall. Music is a useful tool in providing an artistic approach to understanding the grieving process, and it has therapeutic benefits as well. As always, if you believe you are having trouble coping with the diagnosis of cancer or other life stressor, please contact your physician or caregiver immediately.

CHAPTER 6

Lessons with the Professor: A Four-Step Artistic Approach to Fighting Cancer

Nimesh P. Nagarsheth, MD

This book is largely inspired by the thoughts and ideas of Professor Emeritus Jim Latimer from the University of Wisconsin–Madison School of Music. Recognized as one of the world's leading academic percussionists, Professor Latimer has experienced life through the eyes and ears of a musical genius. From his unique vantage point, Professor Latimer has applied the lessons of music to everyday life and has developed an understanding of people that could only be achieved through this deep understanding of the arts. As a student of Professor Latimer's and a practicing cancer surgeon, I have been able to integrate this knowledge obtained from the arts to help improve the quality of life of my cancer patients. The same time-tested and proven four-step approach to discovering the arts as taught by Professor Latimer for decades has also proven to be an invaluable approach in my practice for helping cancer patients cope with their disease.

In this chapter, you will be provided with a practical approach to dealing with cancer as adapted from the four fundamental components of lessons in music: sight reading studies, repertoire studies, improvisation studies, and exploratory studies. The reason that this approach works so well in developing a better understanding of life with cancer is that these four areas of concentration are simply a natural reflection of what happens in everyday life.

Sight Reading Studies

I realize that you may have just been diagnosed with cancer, and that all too often this diagnosis hits without warning. Like so many others afflicted from this disease, you may have discovered the sobering truth that there is no way to prepare for something like this diagnosis. How are you and your family going to get through it? Following an artistic approach similar to that taught in sight reading studies in music can provide you with structure and comfort when dealing with the shock of the initial news.

Sight reading is the terminology that describes the situation when a musician is asked to play a piece of music on the spot without any preparation or previous knowledge of the piece. While this is often an exercise that musicians practice in the rehearsal studio, the goal is to be able to handle this task in a live performance should the occasion arise. In practical terms, sight reading studies train the musician to formulate a thoughtful response to situations requiring immediate reaction.

Sight reading studies prepare the performer for the unexpected. So how do musicians tackle the task of having to read a piece of music and perform with little or no preparation? First, if time permits, musicians look over the piece in its entirety and gain as much familiarity with music as possible. Musicians greatly benefit from taking a moment to **educate** themselves about the overall structure of the piece before playing it.

> Educate yourself about your disease. Knowledge is power!

As part of sight reading, musicians typically run through the piece mentally, imagining what it would be like to play the part and specifically focusing on the areas that may be troublesome as well as on the transitions. Once they have started playing the piece, one technique that is particularly useful is to anticipate what is coming ahead, while staying focused on playing what is directly in front of them. In the initial chaos of it all, mistakes may be made. (Techniques for dealing with mistakes are discussed in Chapter 9.) Ultimately, if little or no time is given to review the piece, they are forced to move forward. In music as in life, time is continuously moving.

> Don't worry about making mistakes right now. You have more important things to occupy your time!

As a cancer patient, you can benefit from applying the techniques of sight reading when adjusting to your new diagnosis. First, get a handle on what the diagnosis means to you. Take the time to learn more about your disease. Educating yourself about your diagnosis is the first step in understanding what lies ahead. Just as in other aspects of life, knowledge is power. Taking a more active role in learning about your cancer will better prepare you for the future, and can greatly reduce the fear and trepidation that comes with uncertainty regarding the road ahead.

One easy way to get started is to familiarize yourself with the short- and long-term side effects and the goals of the different treatment options that are available to you when beginning the process of treatment planning.

Just as the musician can benefit from identifying the difficult transitions in a piece of music when sight reading, you can benefit from identifying difficult transitions in your care early on. If you require a multimodality approach to fight your cancer, you may have to deal with difficult transitions involving any sequence or combination of chemotherapy, radiation therapy, and surgical treatments. Anticipating these transitions can go a long way in terms of keeping things together during this difficult time. For example, at what point after surgery will your doctor start radiation therapy? Or, will you have a break between completing chemotherapy and undergoing surgery? Preparation is key and can be extremely valuable in smoothing out any potential rough patches on the road to recovery. Importantly, transitions are not necessarily related to changes in treatment modalities, but also can be related to getting through a single mode of treatment. For instance, your doctor may prescribe a different dosing for each cycle of chemotherapy in a planned six- to eight-cycle regimen. Knowing how the dosing will be changing from cycle to cycle can be valuable information and help you with your own mental and physical preparation. In this situation, a stronger dose might alert you to the potential of experiencing more side effects. A review of specific treatment modalities along with important questions to ask your physician about your treatment plan is detailed in Chapter 10.

Finally, although sight reading in music is all about preparing for the future, musicians perform in the present. While this statement may sound obvious, it is easy to get ahead of yourself if you are not careful. As a cancer patient, being overly focused on the future can get in the way of your ability to live and enjoy your everyday life. Even more, your support group may also fall into this tempting futuristic time warp, and when this happens the resulting momentum that ensues can be overwhelming. Like a freight train roaring down the tracks, once headed in this direction it can be very difficult to slow down or reverse.

> Find the proper balance early on in your treatment that will allow you to continue to enjoy every day in the present while still planning ahead for the future.

Repertoire Studies

In music, *repertoire* refers to the complete lists of musical works a person is ready to perform, and can be likened to a daily routine of sorts. In an ideal setting, the student is continuously adding to his or her repertoire with each music lesson. In life, holding onto the knowledge you have learned serves as the foundation to successfully build your repertoire for the future. As a cancer patient, you will be pulled in many different directions, and your goal will be to hold onto your repertoire (your daily routines and knowledge base including your memories, concentration, and ability to think clearly).

> Practice holding onto your daily routines.

Musicians take comfort in their repertoire. This is a place where they excel as they have practiced the songs in their repertoire over and over again to a point of perfection. Based on familiarity, the repertoire becomes a place of sanctuary. But one's repertoire does not magically appear overnight. To build one's repertoire requires discipline, repetition, and practice. Discipline is required because it takes effort and energy to work on these parts. Repetition is needed to provide a foundation for familiarity and is critical in solidifying ideas and creating a smooth performance. Finally, practice is important because unless someone possesses superhuman talents, there is no substitute for practice. In fact, a common joke on the streets in NYC is one musician asking another, "How do I get to the world famous Carnegie Hall where only the top musicians are invited to play?" Instead of giving street directions, the musician answers, "Why of course . . . practice, practice, practice!" Although a joke, the truth of the matter is that practicing is essential to improving one's skill set and holding onto one's knowledge base. We have spent our whole lives accumulating our repertoire of life experiences; these are the people we have interacted with, places we have visited, and memories we have created. The patient who has been diagnosed with cancer can easily fall into a poor mental state and subsequently begin to lose parts of his or her repertoire. Having to face the harsh reality of cancer treatment and potential outcomes can wipe away the motivational drive from anyone, no matter how accomplished or disciplined. The goal thus must be to stay focused and hold onto your repertoire.

> **Repertoires in Medicine**
>
> *See one, do one, teach one* is a common phrase heard in the hospital and refers to a trainee's ability to learn and perform a new procedure. Surgical trainees are constantly building their repertoire of procedures that they will eventually perform once they have completed their training and are out in the real world. Although the "see one, do one, teach one" phrase is more of a joke than a reality, there is some truth to this because surgical procedures are known to have learning curves. It has been well-documented that when a surgeon learns a new procedure, his or her comfort level and ability to successfully perform that procedure without complication increases with the number of procedures performed. This learning curve usually plateaus after the surgeon has performed a certain number of procedures, at which point he or she will hold that procedure in his or her repertoire. The surgeon, just as the musician, must constantly work to maintain his or her repertoire.

As a cancer patient, successfully holding on to your repertoire (your memories, ability to think clearly, and other important brain functions) could very well be the best way to stay focused and remain in your comfort zone. In addition, there might be some therapeutic benefits to successfully holding onto your repertoire, such as in the prevention and treatment of a process called chemobrain.

What is chemobrain? *Chemobrain* is a term that has been used to describe the cognitive side effects that have been associated with chemotherapy and include unclear thinking, lack of concentration, decreased attention span, and short-term memory loss. Although cancer patients have been complaining of these symptoms for over 30 years, physicians have only begun to systematically research this issue in the past few years.

Part of the problem with understanding the process of chemobrain is filtering out the many other confounding factors that could be at play in these patients. For example, depression and other medical problems can contribute to cognitive deficits. Nonetheless, a recent report estimated that 14% to 85% of cancer patients are affected by chemobrain, and stated that this phenomenon has become a critical quality of life concern for cancer survivors. The research on chemobrain is still in its infancy, however. A recent study showed that newly diagnosed cancer patients undergoing cognitive testing prior to starting chemotherapy had significantly lower function than patients without invasive cancer. This implies that something related to cancer itself may be responsible for the symptoms of chemobrain, and some have even suggested changing the terminology to "cancer brain" to reflect this observation. Because the exact mechanism of what causes chemobrain is still unknown, there is no standard treatment available. Some potential medicines that are being investigated include those that are used in treating dementia and other brain disorders, but these are not routinely being employed to treat chemobrain as their benefits remain unproven. Until we have a better understanding of this process, experts have advocated techniques such as exercising the brain and holding onto your repertoire as being the best prevention and treatment strategies to fight this disease. Dr. Robert Ferguson, a leader of a team of researchers studying cognitive rehabilitation in cancer patients, summarizes this concept: "If you treat the brain as a mental muscle and exercise it, these functions will improve."

In my practice, I encourage patients (and their families) to hold onto the structure and routine that they had in their life prior to their diagnosis as much as possible. This applies to both mental and physical (exercise) routines. Although lifestyle changes are inevitable when cancer is diagnosed (such as the need to undergo surgery, chemotherapy, and/or radiation therapy), I encourage patients to pursue the basic life activities that make them happy and comfortable. Holding onto things in life that are familiar will provide a source of stability during this difficult time.

> Make an outline of your daily routine (both mental and physical) before you were diagnosed with cancer and try to stick to that routine as much as possible. Do not allow cancer to disrupt the things in your life that give you comfort.

In terms of physical activity, one strategy I have found particularly successful with my patients who may be feeling weaker (due to the effects of cancer or their cancer treatment) is to substitute more strenuous activities with less strenuous activities. For example, if you were running three times per week prior to your diagnosis and/or treatment, consider walking three times a week for the same amount of time. As you build your strength, slowly incorporate running into your activity schedule.

In terms of mental activity, whenever possible push yourself to actively use your mind. For instance, instead of passively watching television, consider more interactive puzzles, word games (such as a daily crossword puzzle), or even video games. Exercising the mind and the body will help you to remain healthy.

Improvisation Studies

Improvisation is the process in which musicians explore ideas and express themselves through the creation of music. In the comfort of a rehearsal studio, improvisation studies are an important part of the music lesson and allow the musician to become comfortable with the concept of playing a solo. In the setting of a band, improvisation typically gives musicians an opportunity to solo one performer at a time during a song. The solo is where musicians shine—where musicians show the audience their musical skills (chops) and create feelings that reflect their mood (or the mood they would like to convey). In this sense, the solo is a form of communication between the individual performer and the band, and the performer and the audience. Soloing therefore requires spontaneity, creativity, and freedom of speech. The field of jazz is based on this concept of having individual players solo (improvise) throughout the song (the history and concepts of jazz are discussed in Chapter 4). Here I would like to focus on how you as a cancer patient can benefit from incorporating improvisation in your daily life.

Cancer patients are constantly being faced with limitations and restrictions, many of which are related to their disease and treatment plan. Remaining creative during cancer treatments, which may include surgery, chemotherapy (including targeted therapies), and/or radiation therapy, can be a challenge to say the least. For example, patients undergoing surgery may require significant inpatient hospital stays, and even when recovered patients may have limitations on activities (such as no heavy lifting or no sexual intercourse) to allow for proper healing of the surgical wounds. Patients receiving chemotherapy can face limitations due to the administration of the drugs themselves, reactions to medications, and other related causes. In addition, certain chemotherapy protocols may require frequent overnight hospital stays, or frequent outpatient visits to the infusion center. Some of the more common side effects of chemotherapy—including nausea, vomiting, hair loss, dehydration, nerve injury, and others—can result in a significant decrease in the patient's quality of life. Finally, radiation therapy can be prescribed in many different ways, but often requires daily treatment at a facility for several weeks at a time. Radiation implants also may be prescribed and their invasive nature may be difficult to tolerate by some patients. Radiation therapy has well-described short- and long-term side effects that can be particularly unpleasant and debilitating for patients. These side effects include skin reactions and significant toxicities to other nearby organs that lie in close proximity to the area being treated. Fortunately, advances in medicine including improvements in surgical techniques, better medications, and more accurate radiation therapy machines and dosing regimens have addressed many of the more severe side effects outlined above, and the majority of patients are now able to tolerate treatments with minimal long-term consequences.

Why review these side effects? This is not to scare you, but instead is to encourage you to remain mentally creative and fresh in your thinking and overall outlook despite the fact that you may lose some freedom due to the limitations and restrictions as a result of your treatment and/or disease. Creative thinking (improvisation) is a different process than holding onto your repertoire. Improvisation is about freely expressing yourself and keeping spontaneity in your life. Therefore, as you read through this book, think of the jazz musician and how your solo might sound as you experience life with cancer. Find ways to express yourself that allow you to remain productive and energized during this tough time. Use this opportunity to communicate with family members, friends, and support groups. Find ways to channel your energy into productive projects, and remember, your solo is your own creation and there is no right or wrong way to play your solo. Just be yourself and express yourself freely.

What does your solo sound like?

Exploratory Studies

In music, exploratory studies refer to the exercises that challenge the conventional. Musicians are constantly attempting to find ways to bring in new ideas and thoughts to push the boundaries of music and discover that next big thing to hit the airwaves and reach new audiences.

Try and try again is the key. Not everything will work, but without exploring new avenues, progress will never be made. When a new song comes out, it is put to the test and the public ultimately decides which songs will make it and which do not. In a sense, this is the same process a new procedure or medication must go through to determine whether it is effective or not—that is, a clinical trial.

What is a clinical trial? A *clinical trial* is a study in the field of medicine in which patients voluntarily participate to test new methods of prevention, screening, diagnosis, or treatment of disease. As a cancer patient, you may be eligible to participate in a clinical trial. Some patients express concern that enrolling in a cancer trial means they may receive no treatment at all, but this is not true. In reality, patients in clinical trials receive either the standard of care treatment (the currently accepted treatment), or a new, possibly more effective treatment.

In the United States, only about 5% of cancer patients participate in clinical trials. In 2003, a study looked at public attitudes toward participation in cancer clinical trials. The authors concluded that the main problem with getting patients to participate in clinical trials was not convincing patients of the benefits, but rather it was because trials were not accessible to patients (or for some reason the patients did not qualify for the study). Another important reason patients were not enrolling was that some doctors were reluctant to encourage patients to join the trial. In 2005, results of a survey were presented by the Coalition of Cancer Cooperative Groups and Northwestern University looking at the awareness and attitudes of cancer survivors toward clinical trials. This study reported that only 9% of patients with cancer were ever made aware of their ability to participate in a clinical trial that may offer them a new, more effective treatment. Importantly, awareness varied based on the type of cancer; for example, 26% of leukemia patients were made aware of trials versus only 5% of gynecologic cancer patients. When cancer survivors were asked if they were satisfied with their clinical experience on a trial, they responded with overwhelmingly positive responses. Ninety-seven percent of patients felt they were fully informed about the risks and benefits of the trial, and 96% of patients felt they were treated with dignity and respect on the trial. Probably the most convincing statistic was that 91% of patients would recommend a trial to other potential volunteers.

The bottom line is that clinical trials are a good thing, and are just one of the many ways you can actively get involved in the fight against cancer and help make a difference in people's lives for years to come. Participate in trials when you can, and take pride in knowing you are helping to keep medicine and cancer research moving forward.

Before you consider enrolling in a clinical trial, take the time to understand the process. Doctors have spent years developing this foreign language of clinical trials and all too often the patient is left in the dark, not quite understanding what the different trials represent or are designed to test. Learning the lingo may help you understand what trial best suits your needs. In general, there are three different kinds of clinical trials. They are known as phase I, phase II, and phase III trials (or studies).

Phase I studies are performed when new drugs need to be tested. The primary goal of a phase I study is to determine the tolerable dose and schedule of the medication. Phase II studies are performed to determine how effective a new drug may be. The primary goal of a phase II study is to determine which drugs should be studied further in a phase III study. Phase III studies are performed to compare the new drug against the standard of care drug. The primary goal of a phase III study is to determine whether the new drug has any benefits over drugs that are already being used to treat the cancer.

For more information on clinical trials, visit www.cancertrialshelp.org or www.cancer.org.

Conclusion

In summary, the lessons of music reflect the lessons of life, and have withstood the test of time. As a patient, you can benefit from familiarizing yourself with the structure, knowledge, and skill sets developed through the teachings of music, and applying these concepts to your life as you move forward in your fight against cancer.

CHAPTER 7

Lessons in Music Communication: The Woodblock Example, Your Sense of Self, and the Power of Listening in Your Life with Cancer

Nimesh P. Nagarsheth, MD

You may be wondering, "What can music teach me about communication, and why does this matter to me at this point in my life?" To begin with, by now you are familiar with the fact that music embodies many facets of communication, including self expression and the free exchange of thoughts and ideas. What is often overlooked, however, is that musical communication functions at a much more personal level as well, involving interactions between teachers and students, artists and their colleagues, and performers and listeners. Because cancer has a way of putting an undue amount of strain on your personal and professional relationships, now more than ever it is essential for you to effectively share and exchange important thoughts and ideas with others, and express your needs, fears, wants, and desires to those around you (keeping your sense of self). Regardless of your background, exploring the connections between communication and music can help the healing process in your journey with cancer.

As you may recall from Chapter 1, music has been strongly linked to communication in areas such as calling, courting, teaching, politics, and of course healing. What makes music such an effective form of communication? As a surgeon and a problem solver, I would like to be able to give you a concrete answer to this important question. However, as an artist I realize this is simply not possible. This is because music possesses powers that on some level are just inexplicable. It is quite ironic: Music, with all of its strength in communication, falls short of being able to effectively explain its own powers. And therein lies one of the great mysteries of music.

Early in my career, I experienced an important lesson in communication when caring for Mrs. Smith, a patient who had been diagnosed with cervical cancer. She had remained in a state of remission (N.E.D.) since completing her treatment when she presented to my office for her 2-year follow-up appointment, however, I noticed an area that felt slightly abnormal and recommended a biopsy of this site. While this area could have been cancer, I knew it was much more likely to be a benign scar that formed as a result of the healing process following her surgery and radiation treatment. Because my suspicion for recurrent cancer was low, I had no problem complying with Mrs. Smith's request to call her with the results of the biopsy, instead of having her return to my office.

A Side Note . . .

Although I always prefer face-to-face conversations when communicating with my patients, I am often required to discuss critical information such as laboratory, radiology, and pathology reports over the phone, e-mail, and other, less personal forms of communication. Unfortunately, this just goes with the territory of having a medical practice in the twenty-first century, as patients seem to be busier than ever and rarely have the time to come back to the office for a return visit to go over routine tests results. Most of the time, this impersonal system of communicating works quite smoothly, and patients appreciate having their results provided to them in this faster (almost real-time) fashion. Of course, as you would expect, telephone calls and e-mails are prone to misunderstandings, and they occasionally translate into a less than optimal situation for both patient and doctor, as demonstrated in the example of Mrs. Smith.

A few days following her biopsy, I telephoned Mrs. Smith to share with her the news that the pathology results were indeed benign (i.e., did not show any cancer). Mrs. Smith answered the phone after only one ring, and after a polite hello and exchange of greetings, she anxiously awaited my verdict. I was in the middle of a busy day in and out of surgeries, and as a result was somewhat careless with what I thought would be a quick and straightforward conversation. Just as I got the words out, "Your biopsy results are negative," I heard the phone drop and Mrs. Smith yelling on the other end, "Honey, the cancer is back!" It was a good 2 minutes before her husband finally picked up the phone from the kitchen floor looking for more information. From my end, those minutes seemed to pass by in slow motion as I helplessly waited for Mrs. Smith or one of her family members to come back to the phone and listen to my clarification. When her husband did finally pick up the phone, I found myself even more unprepared and dug myself a deeper into a hole. I explained to him in a calm and soothing voice, "What I meant by negative was actually a positive result." And as I said that, I had to stop myself again: "I don't mean positive as in positive for cancer, but negative for cancer and that is a good (positive) thing." After confusing Mrs. Smith, her husband, and myself, the only thing that was crystal clear to me at that moment was that I needed to re-evaluate my communication skills as a doctor.

> **An Important Point . . .**
>
> In cancer medicine, doctors use the term *negative* to indicate that there is no cancer detected, and *positive* to indicate that cancer is detected. Of course, in real life the word "negative" has a bad connotation and the word "positive" has a good connotation, so it is easy to see how a patient (or even the physician) can get confused. As a patient, you need to keep in mind that your doctor has spent years of his or her life learning a language that was not designed for your ears, and as a result your doctor may occasionally run into difficulty translating information. So if something doesn't make sense or you think there may be a misunderstanding, you should always feel free to ask questions for clarification if needed. Both you and your doctor can learn from your questions, and as the old saying goes, there really are no stupid questions when it comes to gaining a better understanding of cancer.

Although Mrs. Smith and her husband were happy with the end result and did not think twice about the troubled phone conversation, I was determined to figure out where I went wrong. After all, my intentions were good, and in the course of returning calls to patients for several years, I had never run into a situation quite like this one. Sure, there were times when I had to clarify what I was saying to patients, but in this particular situation, I had discovered a basic flaw in language of doctoring that I had not noticed before. It was as if my whole world was suddenly turned upside down.

I thus began a quest to improve my patient interactions, and in the process I stumbled onto some incredible insights of communication hidden deep in the exercises and foundations of music. Applying this knowledge to both my personal and professional life, I immediately noticed a change for the better (and so did my patients). Because music is one of the oldest forms of communication, it is natural that a better understanding of music will lead to a better understanding of communication. Outlined below are some thoughts about how music and communication can help you in your life with cancer.

The Woodblock Example and Your Sense of Self

Let's begin our discussion by studying a fascinating musical exercise known as the woodblock example. For those of you wondering what in the world is a woodblock, and how is this example pertinent to your life today, allow me to explain.

The woodblock example is an exercise that was initially developed by percussionists using a woodblock (hence its name), which is a partly hollowed out piece of wood that makes a characteristic sound when struck. Today, the woodblock example is practiced by musicians of all backgrounds and can be performed on most any musical instrument (incidentally, the drum set is an ideal instrument for this lesson). The exercise begins with two musicians playing identical simple beats (for example, a simple straight tapping rhythm just like when you tap your foot while listening to a dance song). Then, while one musician (usually the student) continues to play the straightforward tapping beat, the other musician (usually the teacher) plays a variety of conflicting rhythms with varying accents (loud hits) in varying time signatures (different temporal arrangements from the original beat). As the "student," the goal of this exercise is to hold steady on your rhythm, no matter what distractions and crazy notes your "teacher" is throwing your way. If it sounds easy, you should try it sometime (an easy "home version" of the woodblock example for non-musicians is given below). You would be amazed how even the simplest rhythm can become difficult to maintain when someone next to you is playing something completely different.

Three-Step Woodblock Exercise

An easy three-step home version of the woodblock example that can be performed by most anyone (regardless of musical background) is as follows:

1. Begin by listening to a familiar song on the radio (hopefully one you like), and simply start tapping your foot to the beat. Take a moment to get comfortable with the tempo and feel of the song. For the remaining portion of this exercise, your challenge will be to keep your foot tapping with the same steady rhythm you have established from listening to this first song.
2. After you feel relaxed with the beat (your foot tapping), and before the song ends, change the radio station until you find another song. Talk shows and news broadcasts won't work well for this exercise, but pretty much any song will do. While listening to this new song, concentrate on still tapping your foot to the beat of the **original** song.
3. See how long you can hold out before your foot tapping begins to synchronize (fall in line with) the beat of the current song playing on the new radio station you have dialed into. If you have trouble keeping track of your rhythms, perform this exercise with a partner and have them watch/listen to you to give you feedback about how you are doing.

If you find this exercise difficult you are in good company, as most people will naturally (unintentionally) change their foot tapping to match up with the beat of the new song.

In addition to being a fun (and challenging) musical exercise, the woodblock example is also an interesting sociological experiment and an important tool in communication. This is because at its very foundation this exercise examines the musician's ability to resist the natural tendency to conform to his or her surroundings, and thereby encourages independent thinking. The student musician thus learns how to concentrate and focus on playing a part accurately, precisely, and confidently, even when surrounded by chaos in his or her immediate environment. By marching to the beat of his or her own drum (excuse the pun), the student develops skills that translate to the real world, such as learning how to filter through the mounds of extraneous noise and information that he or she encounters in everyday life.

As a cancer patient, keeping your sense of self is key in maintaining your mental health. You have likely been overwhelmed with advice and information from family, friends, medical literature, Internet searches, and elsewhere. Learning how to sort through this information and—even more importantly—how to gently let your loved ones know that you want to maintain some independence in the occasionally dependent process of fighting cancer, are some of the skill sets that musical exercises such this one will help you refine. In addition, a mental version of the woodblock example (exercises in concentration) may help you navigate through the times when you feel particularly overwhelmed by the disorder around you. Simply focusing on remaining calm and steady in your thoughts and actions (playing your straightforward beat) can go a long way in helping you keep your sense of self.

> Of course, there are many times in life (and in music) when being on the same page with your loved ones (or bandmates) is a good thing. In these situations, your bonding experience is presumably something you are consciously seeking out (an active process), instead of something that happens to you (a passive process). Borrowing an example from the dynamics in a band, just as people find comfort in friendships when socializing in groups, musicians find comfort in bonding when playing in a band. Whether in real life or in music, this comfort is derived from people connecting with their surroundings in a harmonious (non-confrontational) way. On the rare occasion in the music world when all the members of a band hit that comfort zone just right, a special "chemistry" develops and the band produces something far stronger and more powerful than can be explained by the sum of the individual talents in the band. When a magical connection such as this occurs, people take notice, and the band will usually skyrocket to some level of success. Chemistry adds depth to music, and this depth is transmitted to the listener in a very real way. In a similar fashion, chemistry exists between you and your loved ones, and the strength from this chemistry will take you much further in your journey with cancer than working disjointedly. Tapping into the energy derived from the chemistry of your personal relationships will empower you, and provide you with an incredibly strong platform that you can use to tackle cancer head on.

In addition to teaching independence and mental clarity, the woodblock example is designed to help performers see the bigger picture in life (or better understand different people's perspectives). The woodblock example is performed in a teacher-student setting, where the teacher is "the distractor" and the student is "the distractee." While we have already looked at this exercise from a student's point of view, let's now consider this exercise from the teacher's point of view. The teacher must not only keep track of his own (intentionally odd) beat, but also keep track of what the student is playing. This is because the teacher needs to know when the student makes a mistake or becomes knocked off tempo, or the whole point of the exercise is lost. In other words, in this exercise the teacher must be aware of both sides of the story at all times. The person who is able to understand and mentally process both beats clearly at the same time is much more likely to understand the bigger picture in life. An example is understanding that the word "negative" has different meanings to a patient and to a physician, as in the case of my poor communication with Mrs. Smith. If you try this exercise and are unable to mentally resolve the conflicting beats in your mind, don't worry. Just going through the process (a mental run-through) will help you understand different points of view in many aspects of your life.

The Art of Listening

In music, there are performers, listeners, performers who listen, and listeners who perform. Among the general public, there is a common misperception that performing music is an active process and listening to music is a passive process. But, as demonstrated above in the woodblock example, listening is an active process and is an important component of music and communication. Thus far, much of this book has focused on helping you better understand your disease process through the art of performing, however, now let's take a moment and discover what can be learned from the art of listening. But before we do, take a moment to consider—what does listening mean to you?

Effective communication requires a deep understanding of what it means to speak and what it means to listen. The powerful lyrics of the "Sounds of Silence" by Paul Simon (1964) provide an excellent teaching example for us to work from. Midway through this song, the lyrics describe a vision of "people talking without speaking" and "people hearing without listening," and by doing so colorfully illustrates the difference between the passive (talking and hearing) and the active (speaking and listening) forms of communication. Here, speaking implies having something important to say, whereas talking implies verbalizing statements that have little or no meaningful contribution. Hearing is an auditory response; whereas listening implies understanding and processing what is being said.

Listening is an art that requires concentration and focus, while cancer is a disease that disrupts and distracts. Does this sound familiar? That's because it is the real life version of the student concentrating and the teacher distracting in the woodblock example. Thus it is not surprising that listening and cancer don't mix very well. In fact, most patients report having little or no memory of the discussion that took place when they first learned of their diagnosis of cancer. While this may not come as a surprise to you, to someone who has not been diagnosed with cancer, this memory lapse is often interpreted as disturbing and hard to believe. After all, receiving a diagnosis of cancer is a life-changing event, and most laypeople would assume that the initial discussion leaves an indelible impression, something the mind records and plays back forever. But as discussed in Chapter 5, the reality is that someone who is diagnosed with this disease often experiences immediate shock and numbness upon hearing the word *cancer* in conjunction with their own state of health. In other words, doctors now know that patients literally stop processing what is being told to them as soon as the word *cancer* is mentioned in conversation. It is not that patients don't want to listen, but rather they are unable to listen.

If you find it difficult to recall what was said to you when you were initially informed about your cancer diagnosis, consider yourself normal.

If you are in a state of shock and numbness in response to your diagnosis, or if you experienced this when you were diagnosed, it's time to rekindle your listening skills. Maintaining listening skills throughout your journey with cancer will help you acquire the information you need to make important treatment and management decisions. This includes listening to your loved ones (those who know you well and have your best interests in mind), and listening to your inner voice (which is a wonderful way to hold onto your sense of self). Listening is your key to successfully navigating through the ups and downs of life with cancer, and this can include listening to music as well.

> *"It wasn't until spring that I really felt the power of music. It was a warm day, and I was sporting my newly grown one-inch grey hair wearing a black and white dress with stiletto black boots. With my earphones on and my tunes a-blaring I was walking slowly through Bryant Park when I got that special universal look from a young gentleman. I stopped and reveled in the moment: my inner 'Sex Bomb' had been reawakened. I had finally found my stride."*
>
> Ovarian Cancer Survivor
> New York, NY
> ["Sex Bomb" is a reference to a Tom Jones song]

In your role as a patient, *listening* means becoming actively involved in your medical care. If you are actively involved in your own care, you will have a better understanding of your disease process and what to expect in the future. Therefore, use this opportunity to get to know your own medical history better. Request a copy of your medical records (especially operative notes and pathology) and keep track of what procedures and treatments (such as type and number of chemotherapy cycles) you have received. Pay attention to changes in your health and the care you receive. Keeping a notebook in chronological order that includes separate sections for operative notes, pathology, chemotherapy, radiation records and/or treatment summaries, and results of recent blood and imaging tests is a good way to stay informed and to actively participate in your care. Update your notebook in real time so as not to forget any important information, and actively ask questions when you don't understand something. Above all, strive to establish and maintain effective lines of communication with your support group and caregivers.

In summary, music has the power to touch people in a way that is simply indescribable. While the secret of how music is able to heal in this incredible manner may never be known, communication must be at the heart of this magical process. Helping to maintain your sense of self and teaching the art of listening are just two of the many ways that music and communication can help you stand up to your cancer. As you look toward the future, I encourage you to take this opportunity to continue exploring the infinite possibilities of music in this regard, and discover for yourself how far music can take you!

I would like to conclude this chapter with an inspirational message from K.J. Denhert, a world-class performer and recording artist. K.J. shares her personal story of how she and her father made an incredible life-defining connection through music during his treatment for prostate cancer. K.J.'s words are her gift to all of us, and her example highlights the amazing, yet inexplicable, communication powers of music.

No one in my immediate family had ever spent a night in a hospital since I was born. Recounted through my mother, an alarming amount of health related information came from television talk shows. This is not always a good source. When my father was diagnosed with prostate cancer, to say that I didn't really know how to react cannot be overstated. Mom chose righteousness as she had been behind my father to have a simple PSA test years before. She saw Bill Bixby ("The Courtship of Eddie's Father" and "The Incredible Hulk" TV sitcoms) speak about the importance of the PSA test and though she was right, she herself had not been to a doctor in probably twenty years.

I asked one of my father's doctors privately how long he thought my father might live with this diagnosis. He said that 2 years would be a very long time since the cancer had already metastasized to his bones. It was everywhere. I remember hearing the word femur because that is one of those peculiar words that got stuck in my head almost in the way that songs get stuck in my head. Also new to me was the term "hot spots," he had them in his chest, spine, even his skull. My father was about 64 at the time he was diagnosed. The factors that I suspect added years to his life were that he displayed something between naiveté and denial, a sense of duty to my mother, a love of music, a boyish charm, and he had some good doctors, who at times seemed to marvel at his asymptomatic ability to thrive. He lived quite a bit longer than 2 years, leaving us about 2 months shy of his 77th birthday. He never spent a single night in a hospital.

We had not been "go to the doctor" kind of people. It goes without saying that we are very lucky. My grandparents lived long lives in another country, and we didn't see much of their aging and didn't pick up any of their wisdom of experience either. My father confided to me that he didn't feel like he had cancer. Furthermore, for things he found unpleasant, he was truly adept at denial. It was almost out of respect for his doctors that he'd try to ask relevant questions when he was with them. He continued to exercise now and then which, for some reason, infuriated my mother who had a vision of how a man with cancer should act. She was certain he wasn't supposed to climb ladders. He thought that was ridiculous and expected that exercising would make things better. He asked to borrow an old rowing machine that I had.

To his credit, he did enough reading to decide on a non-invasive treatment for his prostate cancer that worked very well for about 8 or 9 years. Eventually around age 74, when he was no longer responding to the treatment, he agreed to a mild program of chemotherapy. I decided to attend the visits with him for company, and to help him remember what he was told. We wrote things down in little pads, but even still we really didn't seem to remember much. We played word games in Reader's Digest *and were more likely to remember who scored better than anything in particular related to his treatment.*

The night before Dad's second chemotherapy treatment, I learned an arrangement of a classic Brazilian tune, "Agua De Beber," written by Antonio Carlos Jobim. The song was stuck in my head so I decided to bring along my nylon string guitar to pass the time. The day involved my father sitting for about 3 hours connected to an IV in a beautifully remodeled section of the hospital with brand new Lazy Boy recliners the color of butterscotch pudding. Each cubicle had privacy screens made of a lovely blonde wood with white rice paper. Honestly, it felt like a private booth in an elegant Japanese restaurant. There behind the beautiful Shoji screens I began to play the tune quietly. His little feet started swinging in time, bouncing off the edge of the footrest. He asked me to play the song again. When the nurse came by he asked, "How many treatments do I have left?" Most people probably want to hear "not too many," and in a perfectly modulated caring tone she replied, "Well Mr. Denhert, I'm not really sure but we can ask your doctor."

"Oh," he said. "I'm having such a wonderful time with my daughter I was hoping we'd get a few more chances to do this."

I watched the surprise register on the nurse's face. When she glanced at me I was almost embarrassed to share one of the proudest moments of my life and certainly a defining moment in my relationship with my father.

The next record that I released opened with "Agua De Beber." He lived to hear that CD and the one that followed a year later. On my seventh release, he is memorialized with my version of "Somewhere Over the Rainbow." I say it's because he was a dreamer and I clearly inherited that trait, for better or worse. Another song on that CD, "Man as a Man," was written for him. It's a powerful song that I've only recently been able to perform. He's been gone 5 years now.

K. J. Denhert
Recording Artist
Motéma Music
New York, NY

PART III

The Life Lessons— Getting Comfortable

CHAPTER 8

Accuracy with Smoothness

Nimesh P. Nagarsheth, MD

Match day is a special day in the life of a medical student. It is the day that students from around the country find out which institution (and for which field of medicine) they will be attending for residency. When I matched for the surgical specialty of obstetrics and gynecology (which is the first step in becoming a gynecologic oncologist) at Duke University Medical Center in Durham, North Carolina, I was both excited and concerned. I was excited because Duke was considered one of the pre-eminent institutions in the world for training physicians in the field of obstetrics and gynecology, and I was concerned for the exact same reason. Yet, despite my mixed emotions, the only thing I can remember from match day (aside from having a fair amount of alcohol in my system) is my classmate leaning over and laughing at me. "You matched at Duke for obstetrics and gynecology? You're going to be a surgeon? Good luck! Hey, that reminds me . . ." And then it came, the joke that I would hear repeatedly for years to come, "Have you heard the one about the sure fire way to hide a 100 dollar bill from a surgeon?" Before I even had a chance to respond, he happily provided the answer: "You put it in a book!"

In medicine, specialties are broadly separated into surgical and non-surgical specialties. Although there is some overlap of these categories, in general most doctors will proudly identify themselves as a surgeon or non-surgeon based on this distinction. A doctor's choice of specialty is typically chosen during his or her final year of medical school and presents an interesting dynamic in the lecture halls. In an event that can be likened to the parting of sea, students begin to visibly separate into two distinct groups. The doers (surgeons) sit on one side, and the thinkers (medical doctors) sit on the other. No matter which side of the fence you land on as a doctor, you inevitably grow to believe you are in the right (that is, the correct) side of medicine. Of course, it is only natural to believe in what you do, so this may not come as a surprise to most. But, this self-righteous feeling is just the beginning of a slow and progressive process that eventually leads to students manifesting the stereotypes that have been propagated throughout medicine for years. Specifically, the doers take on the role of the action seekers and learn to move quickly to identify and solve the problems at hand (this way of thinking is often referred to as the *surgeon's mentality*). The doers enjoy the respect they receive that comes from possessing technical skills that only a few individuals will ever know, and portray themselves as deities committed to fixing nature's imperfections of the human body. In contrast, the thinkers are the philosophers of human life holding court several times a day (also known as *rounds*) to discuss and exchange ideas with other doctors about ways to approach and solve complex medical problems. The thinkers enjoy their sense of intellectual superiority and portray themselves as the brains behind the operation. However, what makes the dynamic between the doers and the thinkers particularly interesting is that although each needs the other to survive, an age old rivalry secretly exists between these groups that will persist to the end of time. No matter which side of the coin you're on, the end result is always the same. The doers make fun of the thinkers, and the thinkers make fun of the doers. It is a strange and somewhat inexplicable relationship that works remarkably well in the modern medicine system. Somehow, these two polar opposites exist in harmony and actually thrive by working together to take care of patients and fight disease. Personally, I like to think of this as the yin and yang of Western medicine.

Yin and yang is a traditional Chinese way of thinking that describes the concept of the complex interconnectivity that exists between seemingly opposite forces in the world. I am not an expert on traditional Chinese philosophy, but in my experience with exploring traditional Chinese medicine, I have discovered incredible value in understanding these concepts. The main tenant of Chinese philosophy centers around the fact that individuals are in constant connection with their surroundings on both a mental and physical level. These forces thus exist in everything we do, including music and medicine.

Unbeknownst to me, I had been learning about the practice of yin and yang ever since my first days of college during my music lessons with Professor Latimer. At every lesson I would bring a spiral notebook in which Professor Latimer would document the exercises we performed that day. He would make comments on how to improve my skills and provide important pointers for me to refer back to before my next lesson. Without fail, the words "accuracy with smoothness" appeared in at least one entry every week. At the time, these words did not mean much to me, and I largely disregarded them as trivial. It wasn't until several years later during my residency at Duke that I finally realized how important these words are not only to music, but also to life and to the care of the cancer patient.

Duke University Medical Center is a magnificent facility rich in history and tradition, and walking the hallways often reminded me of walking through a high-end museum. The medical center had been home to some of the academic giants in our field, and the greater-than-life sized portraits of these distinguished individuals cluttered the walls and served as a constant reminder of the tradition of excellence. "In the days of the giants" is the catch phrase that was often thrown around by the senior faculty at Duke when describing the good old days of medicine, and referred to a time when medical training was more like a fraternity than an institution. This phrase typically was used to convey non-empathetic thoughts to the younger physicians and trainees, similar to when a parent says something to the effect, "When I was your age I had to walk up hill both ways going and coming from school." You get the picture.

My favorite "in the days of the giants" story is the description of when training programs had no standard pre-determined completion date, otherwise known as the pyramid system (today, a residency in obstetrics and gynecology is a standard 4-year program).

"You would work for years never questioning when you would graduate. You would stay in training for as long as the chairman wanted you to, until he felt you were ready to be set free into the real world. Then one day when you least expect it, you would get called into the Chairman's office and suddenly, out of the blue, be notified that you have successfully (and subjectively) accumulated the skills needed to graduate. Some people would stay in training for 4 years, some stayed for 6 years, and some even for 10 years! There was no way to know how long you would be stuck in training; you simply had to trust the system."

When hearing this story I couldn't help but think, what if you were a really good resident and the chairman just wanted you around because you were a hard worker? You could actually end up staying longer not because you were ill-equipped to enter the real world of doctoring, but because you were too valuable to the training program to let go. What a crazy time in medicine that must have been, where performance as a trainee was based far more on subjectivity than objectivity. How much of this is legend and how much of it is based on fact is unclear, as the old guard loved to stir up rumors to create that ambiance of *je ne sais quoi*. Definitely, the 10-year resident training program was not out of the question, as for years the Duke surgical residency program had been affectionately dubbed the "decade with Dave." "Dave" was a reference to Dr. Dave Sabiston, one of the giants in the field of general surgery. He authored one of the most famous textbooks of general surgery, and residents would often spend an extended number of years in his program in the hopes that some of his greatness would rub off on them.

Of course, everything in life comes at a cost, and this incredible training experience required residents to spend several days at a time in the hospital (also known as *in-house call*). Until recently, there were no restrictions on the number of hours a resident could work, and as commanded by the senior faculty, the general unwritten rule was the more hours in the hospital the better. However, not everyone agreed that more hours in the hospital would lead to better care of patients, and it took a tragedy that made national headlines to rectify this situation. Let's take a moment and review this historic event that has changed the way medicine is now taught throughout the United States.

In 1984, an 18-year-old female patient named Libby Zion presented to the emergency room of a New York City hospital with complaints of fever, agitation, disorientation, and other related symptoms. The emergency room physicians hydrated her, and she was later admitted and transferred to the medical ward, where she was evaluated by both a first-year resident (intern) and a second-year resident. Still without a definitive diagnosis, the resident doctors concluded that Ms. Zion probably had a viral syndrome and was overreacting to the symptoms. The intern prescribed a pain medication to help control her shaking symptoms. The pain medication cross-reacted with another medication she had been taking at home and, as a result, her health begin to rapidly decline. The intern had been working for over 24 hours at this point and continued to manage Ms. Zion's care with little or no direct supervision. She became busy taking care of 40 other patients in the hospital, and never went back to physically check on her patient despite multiple phone calls from the nurses. Through a series of communication breakdowns, poor medical judgment, and a general lack of care and attention, Libby Zion died within 24 hours of being in the hospital.

The tragedy of this case was scrutinized both publicly and privately, and led to the formation of an expert panel by the New York State Health Commission to evaluate the training and supervision of doctors. Headed by Dr. Bertrand M. Bell, the recommendations from this group became known as the Bell Commission. Conclusions from this expert panel included new rules such as restrictions on the number of hours doctors in training are able to work. Under the Bell Commission, resident doctors are not allowed to work more than 24 hours at any one time, and no more than a total of 80 hours per week. Although these rules had been adopted by the state of New York in 1989, it wasn't until 2003 that the American College of Graduate Medical Education (ACGME) mandated that all accredited residency training programs throughout the United States follow the restricted work hour rules.

Why is this important? In addition to highlighting a tragic story in the history of medicine, the Libby Zion story brings to light the incredible pressure and stresses that have existed during medical training for years. With this understanding, patients wondering why their doctors seem to have lost their humanistic approach to patient care need not look very far for an explanation. How can a doctor be expected to provide humanistic care for large number of patients while working over 100 hours per week, and maintain their academic knowledge and procedural skills as well as balance social and personal obligations? Clearly, the system needed to be fixed.

To make matters worse, work stress often leads to personal stress. Rumor had it that prior to my arrival at Duke, the surgery and gynecology residency programs had been featured on an evening television show for having close to a 100% divorce rate (i.e., residents who entered the programs married finished the programs divorced). Although I never saw any documentation of this television special, the story is still passed on from generation to generation of resident class and remains part of that mysterious history from the "days of the giants." To be sure, I witnessed an overwhelming number of failed relationships during my tenure in residency. Thankfully, I am happy to report that with the ACGME mandate limiting resident training hours (which was implemented after I had already complete my residency training), there seems to be a lower rate of failed relationships among the residents in surgical specialties.

In terms of the residents in my class, the surgeon's mentality had prevailed. So, with the bar set high and the pressure to perform intense, residents in my program were often competing with each other on every imaginable level. Don't get me wrong, the medical teams were brilliant and the surgeons were of the highest caliber, but the atmosphere for those in training was, for lack of a better word, unique.

My unique experience began from my very first day of orientation, when our class was issued our short white coats. What's the deal with short coats? In most programs in the United States, the length of the white coat distinguishes medical students (short white coats) from doctors (long white coats). Viewed as yet another way to keep people in filed in an orderly rank in our residency program, long white jackets were only issued to the chief residents (residents in their final year of training). Maybe from the pressure or maybe from the strict environment, it didn't take long for one of my classmates to crack under the stress and resort to alternative substances for an escape from this reality during orientation week. Not what you would expect from someone about to enroll at the mecca of medical science, but this experience was an eye opener for me. The residency program immediately rescinded my classmates' position before he could even finish his orientation, and I quickly realized even the brightest among us need help, support, and guidance during difficult times in our lives.

Shortly after orientation, maybe in response to the many adjustments and shocking circumstances I was experiencing, I was forced to quickly react and adapt in my own way to my new surroundings. I called on my sight reading skills (see Chapter 6) and quickly assessed this situation as a whole. After identifying the main transitions I would need to be cognizant of during my immediate future, I hit the ground running, constantly staying a few steps ahead (mentally) in order to prepare for what was to come.

However, watching the military-like precision of the Duke way, I felt like a fish out of water. I realized that to survive in this environment, I would need to find a way to incorporate my more artistic side of life when caring for my patients. The problem here was that my surroundings were not the most conducive or welcoming to this idea. In fact, after only 3 weeks in residency, I hit my first road block, and was quickly marked as the problem child in my program. Many believed that I just didn't get it, but the truth of the matter is I did get it—I just didn't agree with it. The story goes something like this.

As the in-house first-year resident on night call, my job was to put out fires. If an unexpected issue arose with a patient (such as fever, chills, insomnia, chest pain, etc.), I needed to evaluate the patient and make an accurate assessment and plan of how to proceed. Night calls were hit or miss. Some nights were extremely busy (lots of fires) and some nights were extremely quiet (no active issues). It was on these quiet nights that I thought I would have my window of opportunity to make my mark. On my first quiet night, I decided to bring my guitar to the hospital and visit and evaluate each patient on my "guitar rounds." Even though every patient was seen and received excellent care the entire time I was on call, the guitar rounds were not well-received by the senior staff. Suffice it to say that the morning after guitar rounds, I was summoned to the chairman's office, which is also known as being called to the blue carpet (in honor of the Duke Blue Devil mascot and color of the carpet that lined the chairman's "oval office"). I'll never forget that meeting. My chairman just looked at me astonished—somewhat speechless—and finally said, "I don't even know how to start." The rest is history, and the infamous guitar rounds have joined the legendary stories that are still passed down from generation to generation in the halls of Duke Medical Center. A few weeks later, a memo came out from the chief residents that specifically outlined all the dos and don'ts of being on call. Some of the highlights in the don't column included no water gun fights and no yo-yos. No doubt this was someone's idea of a joke in response to my musical extravaganza, and I couldn't help but feel that they just didn't get it.

Nonetheless, it seemed that I found myself in several other creative situations throughout my residency (earning the coveted status of double secret probation on more than one occasion), and being called to the blue carpet simply became a way of life for me. After awhile, it actually became a pleasant experience, and by my final year of training, I had developed a special bond with my chairman. In a strange way, we both finally got it. Both of us were right in our own way, and together, we had reached a greater understanding of life and of caring for the ill, epitomizing accuracy and smoothness (the yin and yang). Upon completing residency, I returned to New York City to start my fellowship in gynecologic oncology and my Chairman went on to become the President of the American College of Obstetrics and Gynecology (a leader in the field of obstetrics and gynecology for the entire country).

Accuracy with smoothness is a way life that encourages the individual to balance the tangible (accuracy) with the abstract (smoothness) to form something greater than either could achieve on their own. Performing this balancing act is not easy, and as I have outlined, it can take years to reach this goal only to be disrupted once again due to ever-changing life circumstances. I am constantly struggling to maintain the inner balance that is so necessary to deliver the best care possible to my patients, and to be a better human being to those around me. Music has been an essential tool for me to stay grounded and connected to my environment in all aspects of life.

Living in New York City on and off for the past 12 years has provided me with the ideal environment to explore my creative passions and allow them to flourish. Partly because of the incredible opportunities and unmatched energy emanating from this vibrant city, people have migrated to New York from all corners of the world in the hopes of making their dreams a reality.

As a symbol and constant reminder of the freedom and opportunity that this city affords, the Statue of Liberty stands tall on Liberty

Island in New York Harbor, welcoming all. Not surprisingly, many inspired artists in touch with their environment have captured the spirit of New York in their work. In the late 1970s, Fred Ebb wrote lyrics for a song called "New York, New York," which later would be made famous by Frank Sinatra. In that song, Ebb sent a message to people across the world: If you can make it in New York, you can make it anywhere. Ebb's beautiful lyrics brought to life the intimate relationship of believing in oneself and being connected to one's environment (in this case, New York City). Although this connection may be easier to imagine in a place like New York City, in reality you can find this type of energy and creative inspiration in any environment you may find yourself in. This is because the common denominator behind successfully connecting with your surroundings remains the same no matter where you are. That is, a love for life which is achieved through a balance of accuracy with smoothness.

Simply being surrounded by creative energy thus is not enough, and one needs to constantly strive and work toward maintaining a balance in life. As such, many inhabitants of New York would tell you that the hustle and bustle of the city has the potential to work against you just as much as it can work for you. Like busy worker bees collecting pollen and dedicating their lives to addressing the needs of the hive, people in New York can often get caught up in the quest to advance their "status" and over time lose touch with their artistic side. The goal is not to get caught up in the mundane facts and statistics of life (or in this case, cancer), but rather balance this reality with creative energy and inspiration. Holding onto the arts may be one of the easiest and most fun ways to accomplish this goal. Unfortunately, all too often people lose sight of the balance between accuracy and smoothness, and in my experience that is when the human touch begins to fade.

At 38-years-old, I have been in and out of the New York City social scene more times than I care to remember. When mingling at social events and the topic of music comes up, I typically hear something that goes like this. "What, you play drums as an adult? I used to play . . . (you can fill in the blank with piano, flute, clarinet, saxophone, etc.) in school, but I haven't played since." And, quite frankly, this is what I just don't get. After spending so many years learning music (as many of us do in school), why drop it?

This is a great time in your life to re-learn your old trade, or even better time to pick up a new instrument (or sing). Whatever your interest, learning an instrument can incredibly enhance your quality of life. In addition to providing you with a sense of satisfaction and accomplishment, learning to play music can help you to relieve stress and to give you an artistic outlet to express yourself. When improvising, you will have full creative input in what you play, and by reading music you will provide structure to your life. Music also can provide you with an outlet for exploring discipline and patience. In addition, playing an instrument can be a very social experience and be a source of making long-lasting friendships and bonds that will likely increase the strength of your support network. I would love nothing more than for all of you to join the musical crusade to fight cancer. Who knows, maybe someday cancer survivors and caregivers will join together to channel their emotions and extraordinary life experiences to create a beautiful body of music that could only be crafted from the energy harnessed from this combination of people and events. Of course, even if you don't want to play an instrument, listening to music can be an incredibly fulfilling experience.

Just as a musician must balance the scientific and artistic aspects of music, we must all constantly strive to achieve accuracy with smoothness in our lives. In your fight against cancer, don't let cancer take over your life. All too often, patients and their families let cancer win by allowing it to run their lives. Use the arts to help you stay in touch with your artistic side. Lean on music during this difficult time. Whether listening or performing or both, music is there for you and can help you maintain your inner balance.

So, how do you get started? There is no right or wrong way to go about exploring the arts, but simply making time for watching movies, reading books, going to the theater, visiting museums, and of course listening to music would make for a great beginning. Be active in your quest for incorporating the arts in your life. Find the opportunities that exist in your environment and connect with them. Record stores, although somewhat a thing of the past in this day and age, can be an exciting place to try out some new music, and many will let you sample a CD before purchasing it. Of course, downloading music from the Internet is now a common way to add to your music collection, and has the added benefit of being able to acquire music without even leaving your house.

Picking up an instrument may require a little more work from your end, but why not go for it? Now is as good of a time as any. A visit to your local musical instrument store can be extremely valuable in learning more about what types of instruments are out there, and what might best fit your needs. If you are on a tight budget, many stores offer long-term instrument rentals and/or carry a line of discounted used instruments.

Some other ideas that our patients have found beneficial in getting started include group and family outings at the movies, performance art theater, museums, or concerts. Incorporating family and friends in your artistic endeavor adds a whole new dimension to this approach. Sharing the arts can lead to stimulating discussions and conversations about the event, and can be a bonding experience for all involved. You can create some great memories and share the joy of discovery with the ones you love. Whatever your interest, I hope that music will be an important part of your quest to achieve the balance of accuracy with smoothness.

CHAPTER 9

In Search of
the Missing Chord

Nimesh P. Nagarsheth, MD

In life, there are mistakes and then there are MISTAKES. They come in all shapes and sizes, and some are easily fixed while others may have long-lasting implications and consequences. Regardless of the severity of the error, I like to believe that most are recoverable, and if not recoverable that there is at least something that can be learned from the untoward event. By now, you probably realize that living with a diagnosis of cancer trumps almost any worry you have had in your life before cancer. But, for those of you who continue to worry about mistakes you have made in the past (or will make in the future), I would like to share a few secrets from the fields of music and medicine to help you rethink how you approach mistakes and help you keep moving forward. Your number one priority needs to be reaching and maintaining a state of N.E.D. Worrying about mistakes at this time in life is not productive, and will only detract from you reaching this goal.

Before we begin, take a moment to think about what the word *mistake* means to you. Although a mistake means different things to different people, I believe most would agree a mistake is generally not considered a good thing. For some, it represents poor judgment or a misunderstanding. For others, it represents a more tangible technical error. Regardless of how you define mistakes, what's most important is how you handle them and move forward once they are made.

When it comes to approaching mistakes in life, music and medicine make an ideal working pair to learn from. This is because while mistakes in music can be serious and at times far reaching, they are rarely ever life-threatening. Learning how musicians handle mistakes therefore can be a valuable asset in navigating through the minor bumps of everyday life.

On the other hand, doctors deal with serious health issues on a daily basis and errors in the management of patient care can result in devastating outcomes. For example, in Chapter 8, we discuss the tragic case of Libby Zion and the impact her doctors' fatal error had on her life and on the field of medicine as a whole. Fortunately, errors such as these are uncommon and, through improvements in the way mistakes are being handled in medicine, doctors have been able focus on preventing serious medical mistakes from becoming a recurring theme. Learning how doctors handle mistakes thus can be a valuable asset in navigating through the major potholes of everyday life.

In this chapter, I approach mistakes in a two-step process. First, I apply the lessons learned in music to bring an artistic perspective to dealing with the less serious (more recoverable) mistakes in life. Second, I apply the lessons learned in medicine to bring a thoughtful perspective to dealing with the more serious (less recoverable) mistakes in life.

For our discussion, let's start with the premise that making a mistake could be considered to be a good thing. This is reasonable because in music as in life, anything is possible. For example, throughout my childhood and early teenage years, I made several mistakes during my many live musical performances. You name it, I've done it. Errors such as losing the beat, getting lost while reading a line of music, hitting the wrong note, and even starting the wrong song. As you would expect, I never considered these events to be a good thing, and spent large amounts of time re-living these mistakes in my head and feeling pretty awful about them. But, when I began studying music in college, I noticed something amazing. None of my musical colleagues ever fretted over their mistakes, and in fact most of them never used the word *mistake* at all. It was as if this word no longer existed in their vocabulary. Instead, they used the phrase *in search of the missing chord* every time they hit a wrong note. Although I had not been familiar with this phrase before, I quickly caught on.

In music, a *chord* is the simultaneous playing of two or more notes, which usually results in a pleasant sound. Chords have been well-defined and most musicians are familiar with which combinations of notes sound good together. But music is constantly evolving, and what sounds pleasant to one individual (or generation) may not be pleasant to another. In order to truly advance music and create new and exciting works of art, musicians must explore areas and combinations of notes that are novel. "In search of the missing chord" is the reference to this discovery of something new and exciting through the process of trial and ERROR. In this case, the missing chord refers to the erroneous discovery of notes and pitches that may go well together. Instead of holding a negative connotation, the optimistic phrase "in search of the missing chord" has a sense of excitement and innovation. The musician who is looking for a new chord is considered an explorer on a journey, not an individual who has made a mistake.

The concept behind the quest for the missing chord is probably best exemplified in the field of jazz improvisation, where creativity is encouraged. When soloing in a jazz piece, musicians have the opportunity to freely express themselves. Given this leeway and freedom, a musician may find himself hitting notes that just don't seem to work or go together. In other words, the pitches of the notes may not sound pleasant to the listener. While some may interpret this as the performer hitting wrong notes (a mistake), others may actually recognize this as something new and interesting. Once again, it all comes down to your perspective. After all, one's solo is one's own creation and a form of individual expression, and therefore is very difficult to criticize. If challenged about his choice of note selection during a solo, the performer could simply reply, "The notes I played were intentional and were meant to sound the way they did." In fact, the astute performer may use this musical idea to create a new direction for the solo. This is the basis of creativity and is encouraged both in music and in real life. So, the next time you make a mistake, take a moment and think about the jazz musician. Is there a creative way to expand on the mistake and make it work? Can this error be a starting point for a new journey? In most cases, no matter what the mistake, the answer is *yes*.

In contrast to the creativity of the jazz environment, there are times in music where strict discipline and precision are required. Consider the example of the performer playing a piece of classical music in an orchestra. When a performer plays a wrong note it may go unnoticed or it may be blatantly obvious to the audience and cause confusion among the other players. For those musicians who rely on the cues of the fellow players, one mistake could lead to a chain reaction of events and ruin the song. The classic teaching for musicians therefore is to drop the mistake and move on. In other words, when a mistake is made, it is acknowledged and accepted, but not over-analyzed. The goal is to recover from the error as quickly and smoothly as possible.

In addition, the performer realizes that once the piece has started, there is no way stop time. In music, there is no going back, and any attempt to do so will only lead to further mistakes. In a similar manner, this concept often applies to mistakes we make in our lives every day. Have you ever found yourself worrying about a mistake that could not be undone? Can you think of any more constructive and productive ways for you to have spent your time?

Finally, another classic unwritten rule in music is if you are going to make a mistake, make it loud and make it count. This rule was most likely developed from the observation that musicians often make mistakes because of a lack of confidence. The timid musicians may be afraid to play if they are too concerned about making a mistake. The musicians often will try to "hide" behind the music of the band, hoping that the conductor (or audience) won't notice that they are playing so softly that they can't be heard. But, as one can imagine, the group is only as strong as the contribution of the individual players.

Whether in music or in life, it is common for people to worry about what others may think about them. This intimidating atmosphere, whether self-inflicted or real, can get in the way of individuals achieving their maximum potential. Have you ever been in a situation where your fear of making a mistake hindered your ability to participate in a group or on a team? If so, now think about this situation from the perspective of a musician. Would you have performed better if you hadn't worried so much about making the mistake, but instead focused on the completing the work at hand? Again, you have more important things to occupy your time than worrying about making a mistake. It's time to get out there and focus on what's important in life.

As a musician and physician, I am constantly reminded that some mistakes are more serious than others, and that some mistakes are not recoverable. In these types of situations, I switch my focus from searching for a positive spin on the situation (searching for the missing chord), to looking for the lesson that can be learned from the error. Learning from mistakes is critical in order to avoid ending up in a similar situation in the future, and in my experience probably no one understands this better than the doctor-in-training (resident physician).

Several years ago, I attended a hospital conference where one of the resident physicians was asked to review a case of a patient who had initially presented to the hospital emergency room. The patient had been complaining of a sudden onset of abdominal pain and was in her first 12 weeks of pregnancy. After an extensive work-up including performing a comprehensive history and physical exam, blood work, and ultrasound study, the doctors were unable to pinpoint the most likely source of her pain. Although acute appendicitis was on the list of possibilities, her doctors were not convinced and decided to send her home with a plan to have her visit her obstetrician's office the next day. About 12 hours after being discharged from the emergency room, the patient returned with even more pain and now complained of uterine cramping (which threatened the health of her unborn child). She was rushed to the operating room and underwent a minimally invasive (laparoscopic) surgery. She had her ruptured appendix removed, and both she and her unborn child recovered well from the surgery.

A thought about this case . . .

When initially listening to this presentation, I could not help but wonder why the doctors involved in her care during her first emergency room visit didn't consider admitting her to the hospital overnight for observation. Presumably, if she had been in the hospital overnight when she had presented with abdominal pain, her providers may have noticed her worsening condition somewhat sooner and could have avoided a potentially life-threatening situation. I then quickly reminded myself that hind sight is 20/20, and while it is easy for me to sit back in a conference room and criticize the actions of others, it is much more difficult to be on the front lines handling the situation in real time trying to make the correct decision. Nuances pertinent to the case may exist that were not disclosed in the resident presentation.

For example, what if the patient had insisted on going home because of personal reasons? This, along with her initially relatively stable appearing presentation, may have tipped the scales in favor of her discharge with 24-hour follow-up. In any situation, it is difficult to pass judgment if you were not present at the event, and it is important to remember that people close to the situation may have a preformed opinion or bias that can be easily passed on to others, depending on how the story is presented.

The resident continued his presentation and then put up a slide that summarized the doctors' findings from her initial visit to the emergency room. Instead of using the standard slide entitled "Assessment and Plan," which is typically used in these types of presentations to summarize what the doctor's overall impression had been after evaluating the patient, the resident (making up his own abbreviation) put a slide entitled "Ass/Plan." With a straight face and without missing a beat, this resident sent a subtle but clear message to his audience that the plan her doctor's had come up with was not one he had approved of. Completely dissociating himself from the decision-making process in this patient's case, he went on to criticize his colleague's care in every aspect imaginable (all the while with his "Ass/Plan" slide in the background).

Although effective in getting his message of disapproval across to the audience, his presentation was not effective in getting to the heart of why the mistake was made. Instead of trying to understand where the communication breakdown or error in judgment occurred in this patient's care, this resident was more focused on placing blame for the mistake and distancing himself from the situation. His presentation was a classic example of how mistakes in medicine had been traditionally reviewed incorporating elements of fault, anger, and blame. But medicine has come a long way in the past several years, and the manner in which doctors review mistakes has markedly improved. The evolution of this process is a perfect illustration of the "that was then, this is now" phenomenon, and there is much that can be learned from the current approach we now use in medicine to review mistakes.

In medicine, academic teaching hospitals typically hold a weekly Morbidity and Mortality Conference (often abbreviated M & M), where each department can perform a candid review of errors and complications through an organized peer review process. Traditionally, M & M had been a venue for physicians to publicly place blame on one another when things did not go as planned. As such, there are many stories of physicians venting their frustrations during M & M about how other peers delivered less than optimal patient care. However, around the country M & M has now evolved into a true learning process with the main goal of identifying the root cause of the mistake rather than placing blame for the mistake. Once the root cause has been identified, interventions can be put into place to prevent similar mistakes from occurring in the future. Recently, even sophisticated process improvement methods such as Six Sigma, which has been used in corporate America for years to eliminate errors by focusing on reducing variability, have now been employed by hospitals as a method to decrease hospital errors. With the goal of improving patient care, M & M has become an essential tool for improving the quality of patient care in hospitals around the country.

Applying some of these techniques learned from M & M to your everyday life might be helpful as you tackle some difficult challenges that lie ahead. The most important thing to remember is that even the most devastating errors may have important teaching points. While this may not be much consolation to the hurting soul, taking the time to learn from these errors can help prevent you from experiencing the same pain again in the future. For those rare but real mistakes that seem to have no redeeming outcomes, try to objectively review the facts that led up to the tragic event and identify where the system breakdown occurred. Looking for system breakdowns in the holistic sense (the big picture), rather than in the individual personal mistakes, is usually the most productive way to go.

The old saying, "don't miss the forest for the trees" fits well here as serious life errors rarely occur as one isolated incident. Usually a predictable pattern of smaller errors or escalating events can be identified (often easily in hind sight), leading up to the more serious error. Focusing on improving the fundamental systems (i.e., communication) will help prevent future breakdowns and related situations.

I want you to enjoy life. From here on out, stop worrying about mistakes you have made in the past (or may make in the future). When dealing with minor mistakes, think of the musician in search of the missing chord. These mistakes are simply a part of your journey and can lead you down amazing new roads—look for the positive and see where it takes you. When dealing with the more severe mistakes that cannot be reversed, think of the resident physician in M & M conference. Identify the root cause, learn from the mistake, and make interventions to prevent it from happening again in the future. Then, move on!

PART IV

Practical Considerations in Music and Cancer

CHAPTER 10

Don't Cross the Bar
Without Me

Arden Moulton, LMSW and Nimesh P. Nagarsheth, MD

When I sat back and thought about the name of this chapter, the first thing I did was pick up the phone and consult with my co-author Arden Moulton as to whether or not people would understand how the chapter title relates to the content herein. I named the chapter "Don't Cross the Bar Without Me" based on my years of experience rehearsing in several bands, and took for granted that others would be able to relate to this experience and inherently or intuitively know what this phrase refers to. However, when I tested this title out on few innocent bystanders (otherwise known as doctors), I invariably got the same initial response: "I don't get it. What does it mean?" This was usually followed by an array of unsolicited guesses such as, "Does it have something to do with alcohol?" or "Does it have something to do with boating?" Not having much background in navigating the deep sea, I am still trying to understand the latter. In any event, my particular favorite was, "Does it have something to do about lawyers not passing a test? But, why would a doctor writing a book about the humanistic approach to cancer want to bring in a discussion about lawyers? That won't sell." Once I heard this one, I walked a*cross* the street to *the* local *bar* and *without* hesitation got *me* a strong Scotch on ice.

Written music is divided up into *measures* or *bars*. These represent spaces in time that have a set duration or last for a predetermined number of beats. A *barline* is the vertical line found in written music (sheet music) that separates two bars. Musicians often use the words *bar* and *barline* interchangeably, even though technically there is a subtle difference. Similar to the use of punctuation as in sentences, bars provide structure for the reader in order to help make sense of the written message. In addition, bars provide a point of reference. Like mile markers on the highway that allow drivers to communicate their exact location even when there are no other landmarks around, bars (barlines) can be thought of as mile markers on the road of music.

When playing a duet, it is imperative that the two performers move through the music synchronized at the same speed, crossing the bars smoothly and in unison. Playing together requires a tremendous amount of expertise that includes a combination of discipline, excellent listening skills, and confidence in one's own playing abilities. When I listen to a duet, I like to imagine the two players traveling down the sheet of music side by side. Although a soothing and peaceful thought when there are no extraneous distractions, the duet image can be greatly tarnished if one person is affected by a major life stressor (such as worrying about cancer). For example, feelings that stimulate the fight or flight response, such as anxiousness, nervousness, or excitement, can result in a performer speeding up, and as a result he or she will likely cross the bar (barline) ahead of the other performer. You can often tell when this happens while playing a song during a rehearsal, as you will hear the one left behind scream out, "Don't cross the bar without me!"

All of this talk of people traveling together side by side reminds me of my childhood days watching the television drama series, "CHiP's." The show portrayed the lives of two California Highway Patrol officers Jon Baker (played by Larry Wilcox) and Frank Poncherello (played by Erik Estrada). In truth, I was often teased as a little kid about looking like a younger version of Erik Estrada, and even though he was a television star, I did not get the sense that the neighborhood kids meant it as a compliment. But I digress. The point is the officers rode their police motorcycles side by side in perfect unison (most of the time) along the massive stretches of California highways, stopping along the way to fight crime wherever it arose. In the show, these two officers epitomized the true meaning of partnership. Although possessing significantly different personalities (which sometimes clashed both on and off the camera), together they tackled dangerous situations (inherent to a career in law enforcement) every day. Police officers must trust their partners with their lives, and it is this kind of trust and support that can get you through the stressful times of life.

Nothing survives in a vacuum, and your diagnosis should not make you feel isolated or alone. People have a funny way of expressing compassion and concern, and sometimes interacting with a person who has cancer can make even some of the most accomplished individuals uncomfortable. Trust me, I know this, and see it happen in my practice every day. Sometimes I can't even tell who is the patient and who is the support person in the office because both appear to be equally suffering from the pain of cancer. Believe it or not, the pain of cancer can be even greater to the person who loves you than it is to you yourself. There are many reasons for this, but one of the more common reasons is because of *altruism*, which is a desire for a person to carry the pain of others upon themselves so that the one afflicted with the disease does not have to suffer. Another possibility can be because of a fear of being left behind. This is more common than you think, especially for lifelong partners. A partner may feel that without his or her loved one around, there is no reason to live. As you navigate through this process, do not underestimate the power of fear, and the destruction it can do to one's support network.

Although usually not intentional, families and friends of patients struggling with the diagnosis of cancer can say things and do things to the patient that on the surface may be taken as mean, thoughtless, or uncaring. Often this may be a simple misunderstanding, but sometimes there is a root cause for this behavior. What could justify such words and actions at a time like this? Remember, your diagnosis not only affects you, but also affects all of those around you. Similar to the doctor's creation of a defense mechanism in order to avoid internalizing the patient's emotional pain (as discussed in the song, "Third Person Reality" in Chapter 4), your family and friends may struggle with your diagnosis and create barriers to protect themselves. My advice is to try to be patient with those you care about. Dealing with cancer is not easy for anyone involved and, with patience and understanding, acceptance will eventually be reached for all those touched by this situation.

Therefore, it behooves you as the patient to be aware of how your disease affects those in your support circle. Through gaining this understanding, you will develop the skills needed to lead you and your troops around the bumps and curves that lie ahead. Most importantly, this understanding will allow you to reach out to those you love for support and caring, without feeling ashamed or shy about the reactions you might perceive.

The first step in the process forming a strong support group is identifying who your partners are going to be as you "cross the bars" through this transition (bridge) in life. A partner does not have to be your lifelong companion, but can be anyone you trust and count on to be there when you need them. Your partner may be an individual such as a spouse, parent, offspring, friend, colleague, neighbor, or a group of people with whom you have become close in your life.

Just as officers Jon Baker and Frank Poncherello rode side by side and watched over each other in perilous times, take comfort in your support group. Lean on them when you need to, and don't let anxiety or nervousness throw you off your game. Don't try to rush your healing process (there is no quick fix). Stick with the program your medical team prescribes for you, and rely on your partner to help you through it all. If you hear someone call out to you—"Don't cross the bar without me!"—pay attention, as that person may be seeing something you are not. Remember, today you are not alone but are part of a duet of sorts. And the best way to make beautiful music in a duet is by going down this road with your support group side-by-side, and hand-in-hand.

Now you might be asking yourself, "What makes my partner so knowledgeable in taking care of a patient with cancer?" Presumably, this is not an easy task and being a supportive partner to a patient with cancer is not something that is typically taught in school. Your concerns are valid, and so Arden Moulton and I have chosen to tackle this issue head-on in this chapter by helping your partner get organized and up to speed. Hopefully, after reading this chapter you and your partner will be better equipped to take care of both of your needs.

To the partners, in the remaining portions of this chapter we will provide you with information that will make you a more effective and supportive caregiver. In preparing this outline, real life partners of patients who have successfully completed treatment for cancer provided guidance on what information to include and tips on how to care for the cancer patient during this time. These partners generously shared their experiences to help others cope with the practical issues associated with the diagnosis and treatment of cancer. Each individual will have unique concerns and questions, but there are some topics our advisors have highlighted as being of special importance, and these are presented throughout the chapter.

A diagnosis of cancer impacts everyone in a family. It may be frightening and overwhelming, especially immediately following diagnosis. As a partner, you may experience shock and disbelief during this time, but you will gradually adjust. In fact, many cancer survivors and their partners report positive changes in both their relationships and their appreciation for life. We hope the information included in this chapter will provide you with practical guidance during this difficult and demanding time.

Know Your Medical Team

It is a good idea to become familiar with your medical team before you start treatment. Regardless of the cancer type and place of treatment, your medical team will likely include an attending physician who oversees his or her care. An *attending physician* is a fully trained doctor in a specialty of interest, such as cancer care. Typically, your doctor will be trained in some area of oncology and may fall on the medical side of treatment (mostly chemotherapy and other medicine-based treatments) or the surgical side of treatment (surgical removal of cancer). There are some fields in medicine, such as our field of gynecologic oncology, where the attending physician (gynecologic oncologist) may hold expertise in both surgery and chemotherapy, which allows for a more comprehensive care of the patient. *Radiation oncologists* are doctors specialized in delivering radiation therapy to treat cancers, and often they work in conjunction with other medical or surgical oncologists.

If your care is performed at a major *academic teaching hospital* (or affiliate), you can expect to have several "student doctors" following your partner's care. There are pluses and minuses to this, however, in general, teaching hospitals have a strong reputation and patients can greatly benefit from the close attentive care that occurs when several members of the treatment team are young, eager doctors who are interested in learning.

Your team of physicians at an academic hospital often includes *fellows* (doctors who have completed at least one area of specialization and are in training for an additional sub-specialized area), and *residents* (doctors in training after completing medical school). Medical students are the true "student doctors" and often will be the ones who are able to spend the most time with you. *Clinical rounds* are usually performed twice a day (morning and evening) and can involve a parade of doctors in white jackets surrounding your bed, examining you, and discussing your case. Don't be alarmed; it is all part of the excellent care you will receive.

Other common settings where care is performed include *community-based* or *private hospitals* and *physician's offices* (private practices). In these settings, care is typically given by physicians who have completed training and are licensed to practice in their field of specialty (in this case, oncology). Many of these facilities provide outstanding care. Talking with others about their own experiences in the community can provide you with valuable guidance to determine which local facility might best suit your needs.

The *oncology nurse* is often your best resource to field and answer questions. Oncology nurses are licensed and trained to provide patient care, and dispense and sometimes administer medications. In our practice, the oncology nurse serves as the primary point person for patients and their families, and is a vital part of the medical team. In addition to being well-versed in the different types of cancer treatments, including risks and benefits of surgery, chemotherapy administration and side effects, and other valuable skills, the oncology nurse also is a skilled counselor and confidant.

Social workers are licensed and trained to provide emotional support and practical guidance for patients and their families both in and out of the hospital. In addition, they often help arrange discharge planning for patients in the inpatient setting. Social workers are your advocates within the hospital and are your link to resources in the community (i.e., government programs, legal services, and charitable organizations). A social worker may work with you at any point during your care.

Know the Neighborhood

Once situated with your medical team, take a moment and get to know the neighborhood where you or your partner will be receiving treatment. Make a list of restaurants, drug stores, and other potential useful places of interest so that you become comfortable in your new environment. Becoming familiar with your environment can go a long way in helping you to feel confident and your partner to feel comfortable during treatment.

Planning Ahead for Transportation

Transportation may be an issue for some patients. As a supportive partner, handling the logistics of transportation to and from treatment sessions and doctors' visits can be very helpful. If driving is not an available option, you may live in a city with wheelchair-accessible buses or private or hired cars. Patients unable to use public transportation (i.e., trains or buses) may be eligible for ambulette or van service. Your social worker can help you figure out which option best suits your needs.

If none of these options are accessible or affordable, call Cancer Care at (800) 813-4673 or the American Cancer Society at (800) 227-2345. If you are financially eligible, they may provide funds to help with transportation.

Determining Special Housing Needs

Certain hospitals and institutions have overnight housing options available for families if you are traveling a significant distance to receive your treatment. Keeping your support network together is critical in times of stress, and can help with the healing process. Other charities, such as the Ronald McDonald House, have recognized the importance of keeping families together when one member is ill, and may be able to provide housing for families that need it when traveling is required for treatment.

What You as a Caregiver Can Do to Help

As a member of the support network to a loved one with cancer, you will probably have two new jobs during your partner's treatment: that of caregiver and that of advocate. But it's important to ask your partner how you can be helpful before you take on any role. As discussed earlier in Chapter 6, most patients find comfort in maintaining as much of their regular schedule as possible, and may prefer to handle certain tasks for themselves. As one survivor of ovarian cancer has told us, "I am the same person I was before I got cancer."

As a partner, your work as CAREGIVER may involve the following:

1. Helping to maintain the household. This includes cooking (or arranging for food from friends or take-out sources), cleaning, childcare, driving, and any other task for which your partner requests help.

2. Keeping track of your partner's medical appointments and treatment schedule. It is a smart idea to be organized, and we recommend getting a calendar especially for this purpose.

3. Keeping a list of all medications, including over-the-counter medications, for both of you to carry with you at all times.

4. Providing reassurance of your continued love and support. This includes being affectionate and patient (treatment for cancer can an emotional roller coaster ride), listening attentively when your partner wants to talk (without pressuring to talk if he or she doesn't want to), and assuring your partner that you will take an active role in his or her recovery.

5. Encouraging your partner to move forward, one day at a time. Some people question why they got cancer. Cancer is caused by a variety of factors, most still not understood, and it is nonproductive for your partner to feel guilty about what he or she did or did not do to get cancer. This feeling of guilt can be particularly tricky when cancer runs in families (genetic or hereditary cancers), as the guilt is not only personal but can have far-reaching implications for other members of the family.

6. Providing hope, optimism, and improving the quality of life of your partner during treatment and afterwards. Quality of life is an important consideration for all cancer patients, and as a partner you are in a unique position to greatly help in this capacity. A cancer journey may have many ups and lots of downs. Cancer is an anxiety-filled experience. You can't always avoid the negative emotions and stress, but you can strive for honesty about how you are feeling and accept that the ups and downs are a normal part of the process.

Managing Stress

Stress For Success by James E. Loehr is a useful book for learning how to manage stress. Although targeted for the business person, the methods and tools described in this book have been useful in the medical setting as well. Loehr presents an interesting approach to stress management that seemed somewhat revolutionary for its time in the late 1990s, a time when a multitude of authors and other experts were communicating about how to avoid stress.

After making a convincing argument that stress is a necessary part of life, he debunked the concept of eliminating stress from your life. Instead of shying away from stressful situations (which he rightfully concludes is unrealistic), Loehr teaches the reader how to respond to stress. The reader learns how to harness negative energy and channel it into a productive fuel to stimulate creativity and improve mental and physical health. His program includes a sensible approach of eating healthy, physical exercise, mental preparation exercises, and achievement of emotional control. Although there are many ways to achieve this secure and resilient mental and physical state, we strongly believe in the underlying concept of dealing with stress and anxiety as it occurs, instead of expending undue amounts of energy trying to avoid them.

As a partner, your job as an ADVOCATE includes four tasks:

1. Speaking up for and supporting your partner when dealing with doctors, nurses, and the hospital bureaucracy when he or she needs your help. Ask your healthcare professionals to a) limit their use of medical jargon, b) give you enough time to discuss your concerns and ask your questions, and c) explain things to you so they are perfectly clear. This new world you have found yourself a part of speaks a language you may not understand. Do not leave the hospital or doctor's office until you understand what has been said.

Ask for more information about a treatment choice. You and your partner should be absolutely convinced that he or she is receiving the best possible care. It is very important that you both feel comfortable with the doctor. You should feel supported and unrushed.

If you have any concerns, a second opinion is a good way to feel confident about your partner's care.

About Second Opinions

As a practicing gynecologic oncologist in New York City, I have found that second opinions are simply a way of life. Maybe due to the fact that there are just so many physicians and specialists in a city of this size (so patients have more accessible choices), patients are constantly looking for reassurance that their care is consistent with the standards of the community.

It is a common misconception that getting a second opinion will upset your doctor and damage the doctor-patient relationship. But, as we have discussed earlier, the doctor-patient relationship is based on compassion, understanding, trust, and honesty, and not fear, ego, or intimidation. A doctor who is comfortable with his or her practice style, knowledge base, and skills will encourage you to seek a second opinion if you so desire. Remember, it is *not* about your doctor, but it is about *you* as the patient.

What I often tell my patients is that if a doctor treats you differently because you sought the opinion of another expert in the field, then that probably isn't the doctor you want to have overseeing your care anyway. Doctors are human, but they must be able to control their emotions when dealing with patients, and handle patient care in an objective fashion. Time and time again, it is when emotions get involved that mistakes occur.

Before choosing a doctor for a second opinion, ask how many cases of your partner's type of cancer he or she has treated. To find a reputable treatment center, you may also access one of the following organizations:

- National Cancer Institute. A list of centers can be found on their web site: http://cancercenters.cancer.gov; or call 800-4-CANCER.
- American Cancer Society. This society's web site has a hospital locator function that will allow you to search for a cancer hospital by location or name: http://www.cancer.org/docroot/ftc/ftc_0.asp; or call 800-227-2345.

In addition, cancer advocacy groups are a good source of information. Groups exist for virtually every cancer type. A brief listing of some well-established groups can be found in Appendix IV.

2. *Acting as a go-between with family and friends.* Be your partner's advocate by screening calls and visits if he or she wishes. Tell friends and family what is helpful and what is not.

3. *Making a list of questions before doctors' appointments and understanding the answers.* If necessary, write down the answers for easy reference in the future. Stay organized and keep a calendar noting important dates and events.

4. *Accessing useful information about the diagnosis and treatment process.* You and your partner will likely access the Internet for information. While there are many useful sites, there is also a great deal of inaccurate and out-of-date information that may both misinform and frighten you. Be cautious when you visit a web site; make sure the source is reliable. You are unique, so avoid trying to compare your story to someone else's experience.

Tips from Partners

"Help your partner manage his or her medications. Buy a pillbox labeled with the days of the week, and help your partner keep track by making a list of medications and when he or she is scheduled to take them. Take the list with you for all doctors' appointments."

Tips from Patients

"More than anything, I just want you to listen, really listen. I do not expect you to fix my cancer, but I need to vent."

"One of the worst things is feeling a loss of control. Please allow me control over other things, like decisions about treatment, how to tell people, what to eat, and how much to exercise."

Treatments

Treatments for cancer are individualized for each patient and cancer type, and it would be impossible to summarize all the treatment possibilities for all the disease sites in a book of this nature. With that said, your treatment will largely depend on how advanced and/ or aggressive your disease is when it is discovered as well as your general health and ability to tolerate and benefit from the available treatments.

After the diagnostic tests are completed, your doctor typically will recommend one or more treatment choices. The three most common treatment options you will encounter for cancer are surgery, chemo-therapy, and radiation therapy. Some patients will be advised to have one kind of treatment; other patients may receive a combination of two or all three, or different treatments all together. Whatever treat-ment options are recommended, take the time to understand the purpose of each treatment and the possible side effects associated with it.

Surgery

The mainstay of treatment for many solid (hard) tumors is surgery to remove the cancer and to determine whether or not the cancer has spread. Surgery is not an exact science, and there are risks and benefits to any procedure doctors perform on patients. Most hospi-tals use a standard *consent form* for surgical procedures whether it involves surgery on your brain or surgery on your toe (or anywhere in between). Standard risks from surgery typically include bleeding, infection, and damage to nearby organs. Unfortunately, on the rare occasion, patients may experience severe complications or even death. Anesthesia has its own risk, but that risk is generally very small.

While all of this may sound scary or even overwhelming, the truth of the matter is that surgery is a very safe practice in the 21st century. If your doctor is recommending surgery, he or she has likely explained to you that the benefits of surgery far outweigh the risks in your particular case. In any event, before undergoing any surgical proce-dure, make sure you understand the full extent of the procedure being proposed as well as risks and benefits associated with it.

Always discuss with your doctor any alternatives to surgery to treat your condition, and strive to understand the advantages or disadvantages of each treatment plan.

Surgery has come a long way in the last several decades, and many procedures have been streamlined and techniques have been modified that now allow radical surgeries to be performed through small incisions. Depending on the type and location of your cancer, you may be a candidate for minimally invasive (*laparoscopic*) surgery or even robotic surgery. While you are getting the same surgery on the inside, the incisions on your skin are the size of band-aids and because of that, recovery from surgery is significantly faster than if you had a traditional open surgery. An overall quicker recovery period means a better quality of life and includes less surgical pain, less need for pain medications, less time in the hospital, and a quicker return to your normal lifestyle. Minimally invasive surgery is not for everyone, but is worth asking your doctor about, especially if you are undergoing any type of abdominal or pelvic surgery.

Chemotherapy

Chemotherapy drugs are designed to kill cancer cells, to keep them from growing, or to keep them from multiplying. Only your doctor can tell you whether chemotherapy is appropriate to use in your situation. Chemotherapy may be used alone or in combination with surgery and/or radiation to fight cancer. The drugs may be administered *orally* (by mouth), *topically* (on the skin), *intravenously* (through a vein), or *intraperitoneally* (directly into the abdomen). The drugs typically enter the bloodstream and circulate to all parts of the body. Because healthy cells in the body are also affected—including those in the digestive tract, bone marrow, and hair follicles—side effects including nausea, vomiting, fatigue, and loss of hair may occur. Still, many patients continue to work, exercise, and live their lives normally while receiving chemotherapy.

Chemotherapy administration has improved significantly over the past few decades, and overall patients are now tolerating treatments better than ever before. We cannot emphasize this point enough. All too often patients will express concerns about receiving chemotherapy because they had witnessed a family member or friend experience terrible side effects from chemotherapy in the past. If this is something that you can relate to, it is important to remember that human beings are complex, and everyone is different. One person's experience with chemotherapy is not necessarily what yours will be. In addition, improvements in modern medicine (including improvements in chemotherapy medications as well as the medications available to counteract many of the side effects of chemotherapy) have led to better patient satisfaction in general.

> If chemotherapy is being offered to you, it is likely based on the fact that you will benefit from taking it.

If you still have reservations, one option is to simply try the treatment one time and see how it goes. If you don't like it, you are not obligated to finish the treatment course (which typically can last for several months). We have found that patients who are initially hesitant to start chemotherapy find this approach to be very reasonable, and that most patients who begin chemotherapy continue on to complete the prescribed treatment plan. It is only natural to be fearful of chemotherapy and its widely discussed side effects.

For the partners, being cognizant of this fear and making sure the doctor adequately explains the possible side effects of the particular chemotherapy regimen are ways you can help.

Radiation

There are two basic kinds of radiation therapy. *External beam* uses high-energy radiation to target a specific area, and *brachytherapy* uses radioactive materials placed near the tumor. Both kinds of radiation are used to treat cancers throughout the human body. These treatments serve to shrink tumors and eliminate cancer cells. Radiation therapy is associated with several potential side effects depending on which part of the body it is prescribed for, and depending on the goal of treatment. Please ask your radiation oncologist for a review of the risks and benefits of radiation therapy as it pertains to your specific case before starting any treatment.

Complementary Treatments

Complementary therapies do not necessarily treat cancer, but instead may improve a patient's quality of life by helping to reduce stress and alleviate some treatment side effects. These therapies include massage, acupuncture, nutritional guidance, meditation, aromatherapy, vitamins and supplements (which careful research has shown to be safe), and of course therapy related to the arts such as music therapy. You should discuss the use of complementary treatments with your doctor.

Alternative treatments for the disease itself that fall outside proven, research-based therapies are not a recommended option for patients with cancer.

Tips from Partners

"I think complementary treatments—especially meditation and good nutrition—made my partner stronger mentally and physically."

Possible Side Effects of Treatment

Side effects are changes in the body that are not desired by the doctor or the patient and have been associated at some level with nearly all medical treatments at one point or another. Some side effects are simply discomfort; others can be more severe. Not every patient has the same side effects or has them to the same degree, and there are many ways to limit and control the discomfort associated with them. Specifically, your doctor may prescribe medications to reduce side effects, some of which are discussed below.

Side Effects of Surgery

As with any serious surgery, patients typically suffer from fatigue and pain following surgery. The doctor may prescribe pain medications and other treatments, and the body's natural healing powers should reduce the side effects over time.

How You Can Help as a Partner

1. *Talk with your partner about visitors.* Most patients are uncomfortable following surgery, and it can be difficult to receive visitors. Find out what your partner's preferences are before going into surgery, and confirm this following surgery.

2. *Before you leave the hospital, make sure you have all necessary prescriptions and phone numbers to call if your partner has questions or concerns.*

3. *When your partner returns home, monitor his or her pain medications, and don't let your partner perform any physical activity that the doctor has advised against (i.e., cooking, cleaning, shopping, etc.).* This is one of the exceptions to the rule about asking how much your partner wants to do.

4. *During the weeks following surgery, your partner will need your physical and emotional support.* The physical support you can provide includes helping with meals, driving, childcare, and other household tasks. On the emotional side, being a supportive and reassuring presence can help in many ways. Assure your partner that you will be there for him or her. Your partner's emotions may include anxiety, fear, and feeling out of control and overwhelmed. Being a good listener is especially helpful at this time. Many patients adjust to the stress of surgery by telling and retelling the story of the surgical experience.

5. *Most patients do not need home health nursing following surgery, and insurance will only pay for nurses to come to your house if your doctors believe it is a "medical necessity."* If you have concerns or questions, or think your partner will need a nurse or special equipment at home, speak to the social worker before your partner is discharged from the hospital.

Tips from Partners

"We realized after we got home that a mistake had been made on one of my partner's prescriptions. Double check everything with the medical staff before leaving the hospital."

"The best gift we received when we got home from the hospital was food. Not having to worry about cooking was a huge help."

"The first week after she got home from the hospital, my partner wanted no visitors outside the family. My partner was tired and not ready to see anyone."

Side Effects of Chemotherapy

Your partner will probably experience some side effects following his or her chemotherapy treatments. Because the chemotherapy drugs and the interval between treatments vary with each patient (and individual tolerance to chemotherapy varies from patient to patient), a broad overview of managing side effects is reviewed below.

How You Can Help as a Partner

1. *Find out exactly which chemotherapy drugs your partner is receiving, and learn about all the possible side effects of those drugs.* The medical team will provide education about your partner's specific chemotherapy drugs before his or her first treatment. Be sure to ask for the name and phone number of the nurse who can provide answers to any follow-up questions. Although your partner may never experience severe side effects, it is reassuring to know that something your partner is feeling is not unexpected, but a normal side effect of treatment.

2. *Many patients receiving chemotherapy for cancer lose their hair starting 2 to 3 weeks after the first chemotherapy treatment.* This is often a difficult part of treatment. Especially for women, hair defines the individual, and being bald announces to the world that one is in treatment for cancer. If your partner is a woman, one useful strategy she may benefit from is going to the hairdresser and getting a very short haircut. Then, when her hair starts to fall out it is usually not as upsetting. You can get a list of wig dealers from the hospital social worker or friends, and as you accompany your partner to get a wig, reassure her that she is beautiful with or without hair. Also, you can reassure your partner that the hair WILL grow back when the chemotherapy regimen is completed.

3. *Get directions to the treatment center or infusion center before your partner's first treatment.* Some couples ask to tour the facility before treatment begins so they know what to expect. Get all prescriptions filled. Ask your partner's doctor about the length of treatment and the details on how the chemotherapy is administered. The more you know, the less anxious you will be. Prepare a "comfort bag" including articles such as your partner's favorite snacks, books or magazines, a sweater, and water.

4. *Arrange for transportation to and from the treatment center.* Your partner is likely to be tired following treatment and should not drive a car or operate machinery. Also, be sensitive to your partner's emotional needs. For example, some patients like to be alone during treatment to read and sleep; others like company.

Side Effects of Radiation

Fatigue is a common side effect of radiation, and may not be noticeable until a few weeks after therapy begins. Your partner also may experience skin irritation causing redness. Another common side effect of abdominal and/or pelvic radiation is diarrhea, which is often relieved by over-the-counter anti-diarrheal medication. Patients may experience bladder irritation, which causes discomfort and the urge to urinate frequently. Female patients receiving pelvic radiation may experience vaginal stenosis, or the narrowing of the vagina caused by scar tissue. This can make intercourse painful for the female patient.

How You Can Help as a Partner

1. *If your partner begins to experience fatigue, allow him or her extra time to rest, and be prepared to help with daily tasks.*

2. *Remind your partner to clean and protect the skin exposed to radiation.* This helps control skin irritation and redness.

3. *If your partner is a female who has received pelvic radiation, discuss with her the possibility of using a vaginal dilator, which stretches the walls of the vagina to avoid permanent vaginal scarring.*

4. *Ask your partner's doctor or the oncology radiation nurses for additional suggestions on how to manage the side effects of radiation.*

Tips from Partners

"My partner was tired and sore following radiation. We took short walks every night, which helped with the tiredness, and her doctor told her not to use very hot water on her skin."

"You are going to participate in your partner's treatment. This will expose you to things that will be distressing. You need to be prepared to help your partner deal with possible side effects."

"We got very helpful and practical tips on what to do for side effects from other volunteer cancer survivors. My partner listened to them because they had experienced it themselves."

"Prepare a comfortable place in the house/apartment for your partner following treatment: a favorite chair, a comforter, soothing music."

"If you live far away and are traveling by car following treatment, be prepared to stop often for bathroom breaks. Chemotherapy treatment requires that your partner receive a lot of fluids."

Tips from Patients

"I need reassurance that you still love me in spite of the bald, tired stranger I have become."

Family and Friends

Family members and friends can be an important source of support in many ways, both emotional and practical. You and your partner should discuss what kind of support would be most helpful, and which of your friends and relatives might be willing to provide it. Self-reliance can be a good thing, but receiving a cancer diagnosis is the kind of personal crisis where it makes sense to ask for assistance.

How You Can Help as a Partner
1. *Tell your family and friends as soon as possible.* Waiting delays the comfort and support your family and friends will want to give to both of you—and those who want to help will need guidance about what kind of support you desire. Telling the majority of your friends early on in the disease process also will assure not having to repeat the story from the beginning several months in a row.

2. *Decide which jobs you need help with accomplishing.* Ask family and friends about availability. Make a list and give everyone who offers help a specific task. Some examples of jobs you may need done include preparing meals, accompanying your partner to treatment, caring for children, and reading to your partner following treatment.

3. *Keep a calendar with daily reminders of each day's activities and who is coming to help.*

How to Tell the Children

How and what to tell children about your partner's cancer depends upon the age of the child. You are the experts on the subject of your children, their emotional temperaments, and level of understanding. Be honest, but use language they will understand and reassure them that they are not responsible for their parent's cancer. Tell them that while their routines will change for awhile, you both will be there to answer their questions, and provide them with attention and love.

Tips from Patients

"Before you tell people every detail, know your audience. Understand that your partner's elderly mother might not be able to handle everything."

"Give your kids more responsibilities around the house. It is helpful to the family and makes them feel they are helping their parents."

How to Keep Everyone in Touch

If you and your partner want to keep friends and family informed and up-to-date with a minimum of back-and-forth calling, let technology help:

1. Record a message on your answering machine or voicemail that says, "We appreciate your call and your concern, but please understand if we don't call you back right away. Thanks."

2. Designate one person, a sister-in-law for example, to call everyone at the end of the day with updates.

3. Set up an e-mail group (or a profile on a social networking site like Facebook) of concerned family and friends. Send one e-mail on a regular basis to the entire group.

4. Use Internet sites that let you post updates of your partner's progress. Family and friends then can access the information at any time. Examples of such sites include: www.lotsahelpinghands.com and www.caring.org.

What About Your Sex Life?

Your sex life will likely be impacted by your partner's diagnosis. Writing from a gynecologic oncologist's point of view, a diagnosis of gynecologic cancer profoundly affects a woman physically and emotionally. Recovery from a major abdominal surgery can take up to 6 weeks, and the fatigue and side effects from pain medication impact sexual desire and functioning. Self-consciousness about body changes and fear that sexual intercourse may cause pain also impact a woman's adjustment. If your partner had not experienced menopause before her surgery, symptoms such as hot flashes, mood swings, and vaginal dryness may occur. Of course, surgery of any kind on any part of the body can affect your partner's sex drive (whether male or female) and similar physical and emotional concerns may apply. The point is to be aware and understanding of these changes.

Chemotherapy and radiation treatment side effects may impact your sex life also. Chemotherapy side effects like nausea, hair loss, and fatigue may cause loss of desire. And as reviewed above, scarring from radiation can cause the vagina to shorten, causing discomfort for your partner.

How You Can Help as a Partner

1. *Empathy.* Understanding the emotional and physical effects of treatment will help you find solutions.

2. *Communication is critical.* Share your concerns and fears. Tell your partner that you find him or her desirable but are willing to wait until he or she is ready to resume sexual activity.

3. *BE PATIENT.* Most of the effects of treatment for cancer lessen when treatment ends. At that time your partner will feel better physically and emotionally. Keep in mind that every patient recovers at his or her own pace and some patients continue to experience lack of desire. This is normal.

4. *If you and your partner were experiencing problems in your sex life before the cancer diagnosis, this may be a good time to seek professional help.* Talk to the doctor or the hospital social worker for a referral.

5. *If your partner is a gynecologic oncology patient and experienced orgasm before her diagnosis, she will in all likelihood experience orgasm again.* Some women report their orgasms feel somewhat different but they do occur. The use of vaginal lubricants and moisturizers can help remedy vaginal dryness. Regular vaginal intercourse, if and when your

partner is ready, helps stretch the vagina following radiation. If you are not ready for vaginal intercourse, vaginal dilators have the same effect. In general, you will not feel a difference during intercourse following your partner's hysterectomy.

> **Tips from Partners**
>
> "Be patient. Your sex life will change, temporarily, maybe forever. But with creativity and patience it will still be enjoyable."

> **Tips from Patients**
>
> "Please be patient. I love you but the last thing on my mind right now is sex."

Financial and Legal Issues

Any serious illness creates problems that go beyond the direct issues of medical care—and cancer is no exception. There are medical bills to pay, insurance companies to deal with, legal documents to be filled out, employers to negotiate with, and for some patients, legal rights to be called upon and government assistance to apply for. As a partner, you will probably want to help with these tasks. Social workers and other trained staffers can assist you, or if needed, refer you to outside experts: lawyers, financial and insurance consultants, government agencies, and charitable organizations.

There are a number of financial issues that you, as caregiver, will likely have responsibility for during your partner's recovery, such as health insurance, the medical bills not covered by insurance, and out-of-pocket expenses.

Health Insurance and Medical Bills

If you and your partner have private insurance or are insured by your employers, it is important to review the policies to determine exactly what is covered by your plan. If your partner is not insured, investigate group policies through professional organizations for retired persons, teachers, or any group that either of you belongs to. Determine if your partner is eligible for Medicare. If your partner is uninsured, your hospital will determine his or her eligibility for Medicaid, the state benefit program for the unemployed or those in a low income bracket.

How You Can Help as a Partner

1. *Do not let your partner's health insurance lapse; be sure premiums are paid on time.*

2. *Call your partner's insurance company to find out if a certain procedure or test needs pre-approval to avoid unexpected fees.* Be familiar with the amount of your insurance co-pay.

3. *Ask your partner's insurance company to assign a specific case manager to act as a link between the healthcare system and the insurance company.* This will help you manage the bills.

4. *If the insurance company refuses to cover a treatment or procedure, help your partner file a grievance.* Ask your provider why the claim was denied and then re-submit the bill with a copy of the denial letter. If you have exhausted all options, try contacting the Consumer Services Bureau of your state of residence.

Handling Medical Bills Not Covered by Insurance and Out-of-Pocket Expenses

There will be costs for treatment not covered by insurance as well as out-of-pocket expenses (childcare, travel expenses, medical equipment, meals, etc.) that may present a financial burden. Fortunately, there are many ways to lighten that burden.

How You Can Help as a Partner

1. *Ask the hospital social worker for a list of resources to help with expenses.* For example, some churches have funds to support members.

2. *Some out-of-pocket expenses are tax deductible.* Save receipts from ALL bills and ask an expert at tax time which ones are tax deductible.

3. *This is the time to reach out to family and friends for help.* They will likely be grateful to provide support. If they are unable to provide direct financial support, ask them for help with things like organizing your bills or calling creditors.

4. *Rank your bills in order of importance.* For example, medical bills, rent or mortgage payments, utilities, and taxes should take priority.

5. *If you anticipate financial problems, work out a payment plan with creditors as soon as possible.* Consumer counseling organizations will help you create a plan for paying creditors.

6. *Make an appointment with a financial counselor in your hospital's business office to discuss problems paying medical expenses.*

7. *You can also call your hospital patient representative office for support and advocacy.*

Tips from Partners

"Find out as soon as possible what your insurance covers and what it doesn't. Remember that insurance companies are businesses; they will reimburse as little as possible. Find a health advocate if insurance issues overwhelm you."

"Keep good records of medical payments and insurance reimbursements to ensure that insurance thresholds are adhered to and records are available for income tax deductions. I use an accordion file carefully labeled for easy access."

Legal Issues

You may find yourself helping to organize your partner's legal concerns during her treatment. These may include making or changing a will and/or thinking about advance directives. An *advance directive*, a *living will*, and a *healthcare proxy* (also known as a *durable power of attorney*), allow patients to determine what kind of medical interventions (hydration, feeding, etc.) they will get if they are not able to communicate their wishes or make decisions (issues related to end-of-life care and planning are discussed in detail in Chapter 14).

Most doctors encourage patients to work as much as possible during treatment. For some patients, it may be financially necessary. In addition, work may be a welcome distraction, and a way for your partner to return to a comforting, predictable routine. However, if your partner's doctor advises him or her not to return to work, both of you should consider accessing one or more of the following programs.

Family Medical Leave Act (FMLA)
This federal law provides some job protections for persons who must take time off for medical reasons as well as for their spouse who is caring for them. The law applies to employees of an employer with 50 or more employees working in the same geographic area. To be protected, you must have been working for the employer for at least 12 months and have worked at least 1,250 hours during that year. This law does not provide salary replacement. It does provide job and benefit protection. When you return to work you must be allowed to return to your job or one that is equivalent. You will receive job protection for up to 12 weeks per year, but the weeks do not have to be taken consecutively. You may work in between weeks off, making the FMLA a good choice for patients on chemotherapy.

Short-Term Disability
Short-term disability is private insurance that replaces a percentage of income if illness prevents your partner from working. As an example, most companies in New York state provide the same core benefit: a 7-day wait period, 50% of gross weekly income, a maximum weekly benefit of $170, and a maximum benefit period of 26 weeks. Most employers' process short-term disability claims internally. You

and your partner will not be responsible for extensive paperwork to complete a claim. All employers require a doctor's statement to approve short-term disability. Speak to your employer about applying for short-term disability and ask the social worker for help getting her doctor's written approval.

Long-Term Disability

Social Security pays long-term disability benefits to people who cannot work due to a medical condition that is expected to last at least 1 year or result in death. Social Security disability is funded with Social Security taxes paid by workers. Benefits are based on an individual's age at the time she became disabled and on the amount of time she worked under Social Security. To be eligible for long-term disability, you, at age 60, must have worked for 9½ years. You should apply for disability as soon as you have determined your eligibility. It may take up to 5 months for a claim to be processed. Patients may apply at www.socialsecurity.gov or call 800-772-1213 to make an appointment to file a claim at your local Social Security office.

Tips from Partners

"Speak to your employers as soon as possible about taking a family leave of absence. Encourage your partner to apply for disability benefits as soon as possible, because the application process is lengthy."

How You Can Help as a Partner

1. *It may be difficult to discuss end-of-life issues, but it is important to know your partner's wishes.*

2. *If your partner appoints you as a healthcare proxy, ask your partner exactly what his or her wishes are so you can be sure they are followed.*

3. *Make copies of the advance directive, keep one for yourself, and give copies to other family members and healthcare providers.*

Taking Care of Yourself as a Partner of a Cancer Patient

The caregivers of patients with cancer are often overlooked by healthcare providers, family, and friends. Caring for an ill partner is stressful and difficult. Both you and your partner need support, encouragement and attention to physical and emotional well-being.

What You Can Do for Yourself as a Partner of a Cancer Patient

1. *Make caring for yourself a priority.* Keep your own doctors' appointments, rest, and try not to skip meals, or overeat. Exercise regularly to help relieve stress.

2. *Realize that feeling angry or resentful is normal.* Discuss your feelings with someone you trust, and don't feel guilty. It is exhausting, physically and emotionally, to care for a partner being treated for cancer.

3. *Schedule time for the hobbies and leisure activities you enjoy.* You will be a better caregiver if you take time for yourself. Ask friends to fill in for you at home when necessary.

4. *Plan a vacation with your partner.* It helps to have something to look forward to during or after treatment.

5. *Talk to friends who have been caregivers.* It helps to share feelings and get advice from someone who has lived through what you are experiencing.

Tips from Partners

"Some advice for those who think they can do it alone. You probably can, but will likely not be as effective for yourself, your partner, your kids, and co-workers unless you talk to those you trust about what you are going through. You may need to seek help. Think of getting help from a therapist like getting a good coach. Most of you accept a personal trainer or a basketball, tennis, or golf coach. You may need a coach to help with your partner's cancer."

"I was so grateful to my partner for understanding that I sometimes felt resentful about the changes my partner's cancer made in my life and our life together. We talked about it and my partner forgave me for what I know were selfish but I guess normal feelings."

Summary

In conclusion, as a partner to a patient with cancer you are in a position that is both an honor and a privilege. This position demands responsibility, requires hard work and dedication, but also can be an incredibly rewarding experience. As you travel on the road to the future, always remember that traveling side by side is much better than traveling one in front of the other, and will assure that you both cross the bar together.

CHAPTER 11

Where's the Bridge? Keeping Perspective During Your Journey with Cancer

John F. Boggess, MD and Nimesh P. Nagarsheth, MD

Surgery is all about knowing anatomy. As gynecologic cancer sur-geons, we spent a significant amount of time during our four years of medical school, four years of residency and three (or in some cases four) years of fellowship learning the names, shapes, structure, and interconnectivity between the many parts of the human body. Although everyone knows some anatomy—such as the toe bone being connected to the foot bone as described in the children's song, "Dry Bones" (which is available as a sing-along song on the National Institute of Environmental Health Sciences kids' pages Web site)—a surgeon's understanding of anatomy is no joking matter. Some of the toughest surgical cases we encounter are those in which we are unable to decipher normal anatomy. In these situations, the general rule is to take the time to "restore" normal anatomy before proceed-ing with the main part of the surgery in order to minimize the chance of injuring nearby organs.

What makes cancer surgery even more challenging than non-cancer surgery is that in many cases cancer permanently changes the human anatomy. Cancer has a way of attaching onto things and growing into things that are in its path. In addition, cancer is always looking for nutrition (which it requires to grow), and so it often will make or recruit new blood supplies that make resection more difficult. As you can imagine, in surgery unanticipated blood vessels are not a welcomed sight.

Luckily, we are continuously finding more and more new ways to attack cancer by taking advantage of this knowledge. And, as cancer surgeons, we possess new and innovative techniques to successfully remove cancer (such as laparoscopic and robotic surgery, see Figures 11-1 and 11-2), while minimizing the overall effects on the human body. Advances in modern medicine have made surgery an extremely safe and well-tolerated practice. However, despite the many fancy instruments and machines now available, the foundation of surgery remains rooted in a strong understanding of basic human anatomy.

Until recently, the word *anatomy* had just one meaning for us as surgeons. But, in truth, anatomy can be used to describe the struc-

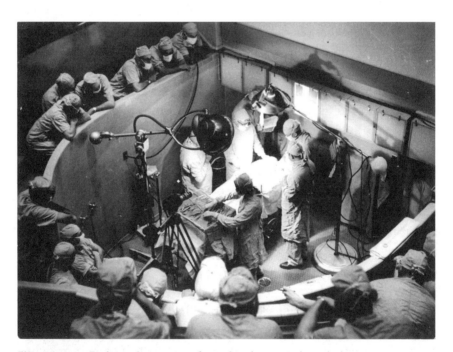

Figure 11-1. Traditional surgery performed in the surgical amphitheater (early 1960s).
Courtesy of the Mount Sinai Archives, New York, NY.

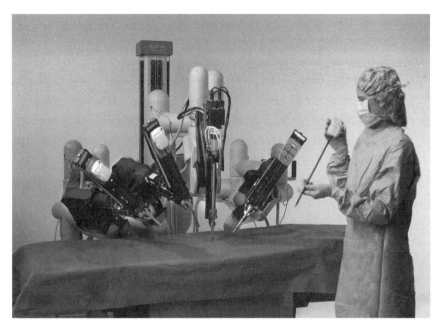

Figure 11-2. Robotic surgery uses a computer-assisted platform designed to help the surgeon perform minimally invasive procedures.
© 2009 Intuitive Surgical, Inc.

tural basis for virtually everything in life, including music. During our recent song writing experiences as part of N.E.D., we stood in awe as our producer and songwriting coach dissected our songs one by one with the precision equaled to that of a seasoned surgeon. Even though we had spent months painstakingly trying to adjust the structure of our songs, in a matter of just a few hours with our new songwriting team, we had learned more about the structure of music than we as band members had accumulated in our collective lifetimes. Looking back on this experience, it seemed that our song-writing coach had done precisely what we do in the operating room: restored normal anatomy.

The song structure of popular music works for several reasons. First, there are themes that recur and provide familiarity to the piece. The verse (often referred to as the *A theme*) and the chorus (often referred to as the *B theme*) typically provide contrasting yet complementary parts of the song. In general, the verse and chorus are the defining parts of the song. Shorter segments of the song, such as an introduction (often called the *intro*) and ending (often called the *outro*), are not always present but can add greatly to the depth of a song. A solo, though not always present, is usually designed to feature an individual performer and brings an element of the jazz influence (creative improvisation) in modern popular songs.

But it's the bridge that may arguably be the most important part of the song. The bridge typically stands out in stark contrast to the verse and/or chorus and, unlike these repeated elements of the song, the bridge is usually only played once. The bridge typically appears after a sense of familiarity has been established in a song (usually after at least two verses have passed), and serves as a transition to link two parts of the song. For example, the bridge may take the place of the third verse and then bring the listener back to the chorus (a place of familiarity). Because of its short and singular nature, the bridge is not a defining part of the song, but is still an extremely important component to its overall structure. But what makes the bridge so intriguing is the sense of uneasiness or urgency it creates during the song, which then resolves into a more familiar segment. In the rare instance when a bridge is purposely absent from the song, most listeners are left with a sense of incompleteness. If the listener is an astute musician or music lover, they will inevitably ask, "Where's the bridge?"

So how does knowing the anatomy of a song help you in your journey with cancer? It's all about perspective. That is, how you choose to view your cancer in your life. Cancer can be your A theme, B theme, intro, outro, or bridge in your life song. If you choose to have cancer define you (A theme or B theme), then cancer will likely overrun your life. A much more healthy approach is to view your cancer as an important, but transient stage in your life (the bridge). As your bridge, cancer is just a temporary and slightly uneasy detour from your life's overall trajectory, and this detour will eventually lead you back to a place of familiarity and comfort. In fact, as musicians and cancer surgeons, we have seen patients cycle through these life events just like going through parts of a song. And, you will be happy to know that after getting through the initial adjustment to life with cancer (the bridge), our patients eventually make it back to a state of familiarity and comfort (the A theme).

Through our own personal experiences, we understand that transitions are just a necessary part of life, and come in all shapes and sizes (cancer is just one of many transitions you may have to face in your life). Whatever your transition entails, taking a step back and viewing it as the bridge in your song may be a good reminder that it does not have to define you.

Finally, it is important to understand that not everything about transitions are bad. Just like a song without a bridge, a life without transitions can leave you feeling incomplete. So in the same way that a bridge adds depth to a song, your experience with cancer is a way to help you see the world in a different light. Remember, it is really all about perspective.

> After suffering from one of the most difficult and tragic losses of his life, my friend, colleague, and fellow N.E.D. bandmate, Dr. John Boggess, went through what he describes as an extended transition period in his life. When he finally reached a state of acceptance in August 2008, he channeled his emotions and feelings into lyrics and wrote the song "She Sings To Me," which would later become one of N.E.D.'s most inspiring compositions. In the remaining portion of this chapter, Dr. John Boggess provides a rare look into the very personal history behind the meaning of "She Sings To Me," and shares valuable insights on how he managed difficult transitions in his life, and how this perspective can help you manage your transitions as well.

"She Sings To Me"

The Story Behind the Song as Told by Dr. John Boggess

When asked to write songs for N.E.D., I consciously thought through what I wanted to communicate through the music and to whom I was communicating. I decided I wanted the music to be honest and thoughtful, yet convey a spirit of hope that would reach all audiences. I also wanted to make sure that the music was entertaining and singable and not angry. Writing a song is a very personal expression and letting others listen to it is even more personal. The song "She Sings to Me" was written all at once over 1 hour on a plane flight home. For me it is a song about acceptance and transitioning through grief and denial. It is a song told from the perspective of the one left behind, not the one who has passed on, and speaks to everyone trying to cope with the grief experienced when they lose someone close. In addition, it is a song that reflects the philosophical/religious notion that the spirit is enduring beyond physical life, and that we are all connected by the human condition.

She Sings To Me (original version)
© 2009 by N.E.D.
Lyrics and music by John F. Boggess

(Verse 1)
Singing for the love of singing
Each note phrased with a spirit for living
And I believe I can still hear her singing
Just for me

Her life resurrected from memories
Pieced together from feeling
And I believe I can hear her singing
Just for me

(Chorus)
Her melody it makes me sing
Her melody it makes me dream
And though her song ended early
I still believe I can hear her singing
Just for me
Just for me

(*Verse 2*)
For too many years have I lived with this silence
Afraid to embrace a life ended in violence
But now I can hear her singing

It's not just a matter of forgiveness
Or coming to peace with her illness
But a deep need to hear her

(*Bridge*)
All children need comfort
All lovers need trust
Without melody, sadness can fill even the brightest among us
And when our memories grow too strong
We can lose our need to belong
I will live without fear and doubt
And listen once again inside for her
As she sings to me

(*Chorus*)
Her melody it makes me sing
Her melody it makes me dream
And though her song ended early
I still believe I can hear her singing
Just for me
Just for me

(*Verse 3*)
As I let her songs fill me once again
Memories of her rush on in
Her spirit brought to life in melodic
Resurrection

Like a song bird unseen from across the canyons
I can hear her voice echoing
My constant companion
As she sings for me

The musical structure of the song is simple: verse/chorus/verse/ bridge/chorus/verse. Each verse ends by referring to "her" singing to me. But, in order to fully understand these lyrics, I need to tell a short story.

I was born the youngest of seven children—six boys and one girl. My sister is 10 years older than me. When I was a child, I shared her room because space was limited and she was the only girl among so many boys. My sister was gifted with a beautiful singing voice, and she would play her guitar and sing me to sleep every night when I was a child. The closeness and bond we developed together became a very close friendship as adults, and my sister always supported me and looked out for me. Unfortunately, despite all of her strength, beauty, and talent, she suffered from depression and at the age of 39, she took her own life. To know that my sister believed that the only course of action she had available to her was to take her own life was overwhelming. I really did not have any skills to cope with her loss and in order to keep moving forward, I just put her memory away.

I do remember that the most difficult thing was the "movie" that played over and over in my head of what must have happened when she died. It is the mind's need to make sense of things that we cannot really understand that is an essential part of moving through the stages of grief, and I have learned from many of my patient's families that they too have had a similar experience when they lost someone close. It is a need to know detail to replace our image of what must have happened with what in fact was real. This is a process of coping that is very important to moving toward accep- tance. The truth, no matter how difficult, is always more comforting than not knowing.

For years I used the hurt I experienced to open up to my patients, and in a sense used it as "credentials" for being a part of their care and having something to say to them when they were trying to cope with their illness or even death. I developed a thick skin and put my sister's memory to use like any other experience that prepares us to perform a task. I can honestly say, however, that I did not accept her death or embrace her memory without feeling sadness and despair.

While music had always been in my life, with the all-consuming devotion to doctoring, I had let it out of my life. Not until my daughter was old enough and I wanted to give her the gift of learning did playing music come back into my life. I started playing piano with my daughter and then started taking jazz guitar lessons. For the first time, I felt that I was truly learning to be a musician. At this same time, my brother shared with me a tape that he had found among my sister's belongings. The tape was made 15 years earlier of my sister singing and playing guitar. When I listened to it for the first time, it was like reuniting with everything that I remembered about her spirit, beauty, and talent. What was not there was the mental "movie" of her death. It was gone and what was left was every warm feeling and memory that I could relive about my sister. I took the tape and cleaned it up digitally and put it on my iPod. I even let others listen to it, proud of my sister's incredible voice and talent. I was no longer sharing her story of tragedy, but I was sharing her life and her gifts.

While flying home from a family vacation to see my oldest brother, I was listening to her music over and over again, and for the first time in 15 years I opened up completely and sobbed while thinking of how much I missed her, but was comforted by all the memories the music invoked in me. She was "singing to me" once again, and the lyrics for a song just fell on the page. When I read back to myself what I had written down, I told her I loved her and missed her, and a new relationship between she and myself was born.

What my story is meant to illustrate is how a transition in life can come in so many ways, and there is no expiration date on when or how it can happen. Writing "She Sings To Me" and forming a new (and familiar) relationship with my sister marked the end of a long transition (bridge) in my life and brought me to a place of comfort. Your transition is still being played out, and I encourage you to view the reality about cancer not as the end of your song, but as a bridge to something better and an important part of your healing process.

My sister's music not only helped me to rediscover her memory and come to peace with the grief I had been carrying around with me for so many years, but it also unlocked a strength in me to better cope and understand the illness, disease, and tragedy that I deal with everyday as a cancer doctor. It is my hope that "She Sings To Me" will help you see beyond the fear and grief associated with cancer, and to view cancer as just a small bridge in your song. We all have a song. That is our spirit, and it is there for all to listen. My sister sings to me "like a songbird unseen from across the canyon, my constant companion." What could be more comforting and peaceful than that?

CHAPTER 12

Either You Is or You Ain't: If You Don't Get Passionate About Your Cause, How Can You Expect Anyone Else To?

Nimesh P. Nagarsheth, MD

> You're either in the fight against cancer or you're not; it's time to get passionate about your cause!

It is a common saying among musicians: "Either you is, or you ain't." The phrase says it all, and believe it or not requires no further explanation among most performers. As if derived from an ancient language with magical powers, these six simple words speak volumes to the performing artist. For those of you who are still wondering what I am talking about, a reasonable translation of this phrase is, "If you don't get passionate about your own music, you can't expect anyone else to get passionate about it." Whenever I think about this concept, I am reminded about the infamous Billy Joel incident in Russia. For those of you who don't know (or remember) what I am talking about, let's take moment and go back in time—back in the U.S.S.R.

In May 1987, Billy Joel made history when the *New York Times* announced he would be taking his world tour to the Soviet Union.

He would become the first American pop musician to take a fully equipped staged show to Russia and the first American rock musician to perform in the Soviet Union under the renewed cultural exchanges agreement, which had been signed in Geneva between the United States and the Soviet Union in 1985. It was a great idea—music helping to bridge the gap between two vastly different cultures.

The *New York Times* began to follow the story closely and portrayed this six-performance Soviet tour as a breakthrough in international relations. Paying particular attention to the audience response, the media essentially performed an observational scientific research study of this tour, with several reports documenting a phenomenon that was much more than just concertgoers having fun at a concert. A cultural revolution was occurring in these electrified stadiums, and audiences had traded in orderly conduct for free will (at least for one night). To paraphrase one reporter, people were no longer following the rules, but they were following the music.

As a seasoned and respected performer, Billy Joel knew how to engage the crowd, and he knew how important this interaction is in making his show a success. To this end, one night in late July of 1987 in Moscow's Olympic Sports Complex (filled to capacity), Billy became frustrated when the lighting crew kept the lights on over the audience at the concert. He realized that the audience would not truly immerse themselves in the experience if the lights were on because the complex was filled with guards and other visible security personnel that had been put in place to contrast the message of freedom of music. In the heat of the moment and as an expression of his frustration, he flipped over his electric piano and banged his microphone on the floor. Interestingly, the crowd was unsure as to whether this "tantrum" was part of the show and was perfectly unaffected. During the second half of the show (with the lights down), the audience was described as enthusiastic with fans jumping in the air and crowding the stage, and even the guards were noted to be rocking to the music.

Many critics have considered this event as a minor international incident, however, there was no major fall out (political or otherwise) from this performance. In fact, the incident was actually celebrated when the electric piano that had been flipped on stage, which had been affectionately named "Trashed in the U.S.S.R.," later became a piece of history hanging on the wall of the Hard Rock Café in New York City.

If you haven't guessed by now, we like to be optimistic in our field as cancer surgeons and are constantly trying to find the positive message we can take away from a story or an event. So, although his actions were clearly unnecessary, the one thing that Billy Joel did demonstrate through this unusual event is his passion for music. And in doing so, he touched the lives of thousands under Communist rule and gave them a glimpse of hope during that night of musical freedom. Four years later, the U.S.S.R. dissolved, and the people of Russia became free from Communist rule.

I want you to become passionate about joining the fight against cancer. Just as the musician must be passionate about his music before others take interest, the support for your cause needs to start from within. In 2008 it was estimated that over 1.4 million people in the United States would be diagnosed with cancer, and over 500,000 people would die from this devastating disease.

Cancer is the great equalizer. No matter where you are in the spectrum of life, rich or poor, highly educated or uneducated, young or old, black or white (or anything in between), cancer can strike. If every patient and their family got involved in the fight to eradicate this disease, we would be able to make incredible contributions in the lives of millions. There are so many ways to help and no matter what your personality or background, you are likely to find a way to participate that suits your style. To simply sit idle is to remain silent, and as a society, we cannot afford to remain silent any longer.

Interestingly, the association relating silence and cancer is not a new concept. Paul Simon eloquently described one of the most memorable analogies of silence and cancer in the lyrics to his song entitled, "The Sounds of Silence" written in 1964. A phrase in this song, "Silence like a cancer grows" depicts the lack of verbal communication in society as a rapidly spreading disease. Extrapolating from this concept, this association brings home the message that cancer feeds on silence.

An Interesting Fact

Although a flop when first released, "The Sounds of Silence" touched the soul of millions and would later be named the eighteenth most played song on radio and television in the 20th century.

Hopefully, you will choose to participate in the fight against cancer. Assuming this is the case, I want to give you a few helpful hints on how to get started, on the different ways you can help, and on how you can more effectively make a difference in your cause.

In my experience, the biggest barrier facing patients and families who are looking to get involved has simply been figuring out how to get started. Therefore, Appendix IV of this book provides you with information (including name and type of organization, contact information, and Web site addresses) for charities, support groups, foundations, and cancer societies for many of the cancer types. Although this list is not comprehensive, it can be a useful guide in to help you begin the process of getting involved. Because of federal privacy laws, your health information is not public knowledge. Therefore, you should not expect support and advocacy groups to automatically contact you if you have been diagnosed with cancer. You need to take the first step and reach out to the groups you wish to learn more about. If you do not see your cancer listed, or do not see the type of organization that you would like more information on, please ask your doctor for more information and how you can get involved.

In addition to participating in clinical trials and helping to advance research (discussed in Chapter 6), the American Cancer Society (ACS) provides an organized approach designed to help patients and interested individuals figure out the different ways to get involved in their cause. The ACS breaks down involvement into four categories: donation, participation, volunteering, and advocacy. We will briefly review the benefits of each of these below.

Financial Support

Donations and other forms of financial support from the public represent a major source of funding for many societies and foundations working in the fight against cancer. Unfortunately, a recession that began in 2008 has become a full-fledged global reality and will likely result in a significant decrease in funding from the public and private sectors for several years. The federal government has responded in part by developing economic stimulus programs that are aimed in increasing the research grants and funding through the National Institutes of Health (NIH). The hope is that these grants will allow researchers to pursue new and exciting avenues of promising research and create immediate jobs that will lead to eventual financial stability and future advances in medicine and economic growth.

Despite this effort, even the smallest of donations can help make a difference. Consider for a moment the 1.4 million people who will be diagnosed with cancer this year in the United States. If each patient and one family member contributed 10 dollars to the cause, we would have generated 28 million dollars in revenue available for immediate use by the organizations this year. Most donations are tax deductible, and in many cases non-cash donations (i.e., donating an old car or other property) also count for the property's fair market value. As always, please consult your tax advisor about your specific situation before making any sizable donation, and of course only donate if you are financially able.

Participating

Getting involved in the fight against cancer does not require making financial contributions. Another very needed and rewarding way to help is through participation in community activities and national organizations. There are numerous opportunities in this regard, including participation in awareness and education campaigns, fundraising events, walks/marathons and other sporting events, music concerts, charity balls and galas, bake sales, and more. Identify your interest, and get involved. Do you have an idea for an event? Present it to your local organization and make it happen. Most charities and foundations welcome new and creative ideas, and organizing an event is a great way to express yourself and channel your energy in a productive manner.

Volunteering

Volunteering in your community is another great way to make a difference in the lives of others. For example, we have implemented a volunteer program at our hospital called "Woman to Woman." In this program, survivors of gynecologic cancers are professionally trained to help any woman with a gynecologic cancer who desires assistance. The volunteers provide one-on-one counseling, empathetic understanding, practical support, assistance with navigating the healthcare system, stress reduction, and guidance on how to connect with other available resources. The benefits of volunteering go far beyond what can be written in this book, and the personal sense of fulfillment that can be achieved through volunteering has been the focus of numerous publications. In addition to helping cancer patients and their families, volunteering will allow you to make a meaningful difference in society on a schedule that is flexible, and create new long-lasting friendships and relationships. Finally, volunteering in groups (side by side with your family and friends) will help strengthen your support network.

Advocacy

Finally, advocacy is a great way to get involved and make a difference in the lives of cancer patients and society in general. Cancer advocates are individuals who work on behalf of cancer patients and their families to influence change and policies at the political, social, and economic levels. Cancer is not just an illness—it is a global public health problem. As such, national and international health policies affect the lives of millions every day and are just as important as caring for the individual patient. Your involvement in advocacy can help effect change.

The American Cancer Society Cancer Action Network (ACS CAN), the sister advocacy group of the American Cancer Society, is just one example of an organization that has been instrumental in helping to implement laws and other policies that affect how you receive your medical care. For example, the ACS CAN has had a strong influence on getting laws passed that now require insurance companies to cover important prevention and screening strategies such as mammograms and colonoscopies.

Although it seems like a given, often times even important and effective innovations in health care require advocacy to bring them to the attention of the mainstream public. A more recent example of the success of advocacy is second-hand smoke prevention and awareness. It wasn't long ago that smoking in public facilities was commonplace. Thanks to the hard work of advocacy groups like this one, several states and thousands of communities are now smoke-free in both private and public spaces.

There are many ways you can get involved in advocacy. Some are joining existing organized groups, writing letters to your local politicians and representatives, and taking on media and public speaking opportunities. As a cancer patient and an advocate, what you say and what you do has important meaning and implications to those around you. You may have already noticed that people who have been traditionally caught up in the perfunctory routines of everyday life seem to pay more attention to your words (assuming you have shared your diagnosis with them). This is because cancer has a way of grabbing the attention of your friends, families, and others. Now more than ever, being an effective communicator is critical.

Now is the Time

In summary, now is a good time to get involved in your cause, and you can make a difference through donations, participation, volunteering, and advocacy. Because getting started is the hardest step, a list of relevant organizations and their contact information is provided for you in Appendix IV. Just like the musician trying to engage the audience, the enthusiasm must begin from within. If you don't get passionate about the fight against cancer, you can't expect anyone else to.

CHAPTER 13

In Music, the Rests Are as Important as the Notes

William E. Winter, III, MD and Nimesh P. Nagarsheth, MD

Have you ever wondered how a simple piece of paper (a.k.a. sheet music) could hold all the information for a group of musicians to make beautiful music? Consider, for example, a conductor standing at the helm of an orchestra looking over a musical score of Beethoven's "Fifth Symphony." The conductor's score has each musician's part integrated into one colossally intricate piece of music. Despite this daunting image, written music is not as mysterious as you might think. In actuality, written music boils down to just different combinations of two simple types of raw data: notes and rests.

A *musical note* can be loosely defined as a symbol that designates the duration and pitch of a sound, whereas a *musical rest* designates the duration of a silence (or absence of a sound). Notes and rests coexist in music as similar opposites. Similar because they both convey to the musician what he or she should be "doing" at a given moment in time, and opposite because the actual act of "doing" is an all-or-none phenomenon, which translates into either playing or not playing a given note. Rests come in many different sizes (durations), and are measured in units of time that follow simple mathematical principles. For example, in the common time signature of music, four quarter rests are the same duration of time as two half rests, which is the same as one whole rest. Suffice it to say, there are rests for any occasion.

It is a common misconception among many musicians and non-musicians alike that notes are more important than rests. This is not surprising as it is natural to associate music with the sounds that create the melody, rather than with the quiet spaces between the notes. Because rests are silent, people often misinterpret these empty spaces as unimportant. But, imagine what would happen if a song was made up of only notes, and no rests. Aside from the fact that the "rests would be history" (pun intended), there would be a wall of sound with no reference point or discernable backbone to the music. This is because the spaccs between the sounds provide a baseline and contrast for the piece, and give music structure and texture. In fact, it is a common saying among experienced musicians that a full measure of rest can hold more music than a full measure of blistering notes.

One of the most interesting characteristics about rests is the versatility they possess in terms of eliciting emotions from the listener. Rests have the ability to create a sense of relaxation and comfort, but also can create a sense of tension and urgency. When perfectly timed and placed, rests become the foundation for the song's energy to blossom and thrive.

Rest Evoking

A well-known pianist once sat down in front of his piano on stage in the ready position for over 4 minutes without playing a single note. Written on his sheet of music was one very long rest. Needless to say, after only a few seconds in this position, the audience began to grumble, anxiously waiting for what they considered the start of the performance. After a few minutes had passed, the audience grew increasingly restless and by the fourth minute the concert hall emanated of sounds and loud conversation similar to that of a noisy bar. At this point, the pianist picked up his sheet music and walked off stage. His piece was over. What the audience didn't realize is that the sounds they were making were a part of the performance. Their movements—coughs and sneezes, conversation, grumbling, and laughter—were the "notes" of this song. Although somewhat abstract and definitely a little bit off the beaten path, this performance is a perfect example of how rests can evoke a multitude of emotions from an audience including anticipation, tension, anxiousness, laughter, and of course relaxation.

Why are rests important during your cancer therapy? Rests provide you with a pause and a deep breath in your journey with cancer.

There may be times during your treatment course when the desire to continue with chemotherapy, radiation therapy, and/or surgery will consume every ounce of energy in your body. While this drive is sometimes necessary, it is not realistic or healthy to maintain this consuming lifestyle for long periods of time. Just as rests are important in music, taking a break will help you feel refreshed and rekindle your vitality.

Of course, the timing of the rest depends upon where you are in your treatment, and just like in any song or performance should be well thought out. You may not need (or want) to rest if you are in the beginning of therapy, when the ultimate goal of your treatment is likely curative. However, if your goal of treatment is more in line with palliation than achieving a cure, rests may be taken more frequently and for longer durations. As with most things in life, timing is everything.

As oncologists, we are willing to push our patients the hardest when there is a realistic possibility of achieving a cure. Like the energetic first song in a performance, we typically view *primary therapy* (the first set of treatments for any patient) as an aggressive attempt toward achieving this goal. In this circumstance, patients are advised that it is probably worth forgoing taking breaks to avoid unnecessary treatment delays. In fact, we sometimes give patients medications during their chemotherapy and/or radiation treatments to help stimulate their bone marrow to ensure they stay on schedule with their therapy.

Similarly, we often will start our patients on chemotherapy (if indicated) even before they have fully recovered from major surgery. In this scenario, our patients may forego taking a break in an effort to get a theoretical head start on destroying any remaining cancer cells that may not have been completely removed surgically. As an aside, it is important to note that this tactic has not been proven, but falls in line with the surgeon's mentality of aggressively treating cancer. Therefore, rests and breaks may not be a routine part of your cancer treatments, but of course they are available should you need them.

> Aggressive therapy comes at a cost, which usually translates into an increase in side effects and a temporary decrease in your quality of life. Taking this into consideration, you and your doctor will need to find the treatment plan that is right for you.

When the likelihood of achieving a cure is low, the goal of treatment will often shift to a *palliative approach* (focusing on helping patient to feel better). In this scenario, quality of life takes center stage with the objective to not make patients any sicker with therapy than they already are from the cancer itself. Quality of life is where rests come into play in the care of the cancer patient, and as oncologists and human beings, we recognize that everyone needs a break to re-energize periodically.

The Will to Fight

Not too long ago, a patient suffering from recurrent cancer came to the office looking worn out. She had been in a fight against cancer for several years, and during her treatment course had undergone multiple surgeries and completed several rounds of chemotherapy. By the look on her face, it was clear that she needed a break, even if it was a short one.

When it was suggested that she take a week off from her scheduled chemotherapy, she reluctantly agreed. She expressed concern that by postponing her chemotherapy she felt she wasn't "fighting" as hard as she could. She was reassured that 1 week off from treatment did not mean she was giving up or not trying hard enough, but rather may actually help her in the long run. After her week off, she returned rejuvenated and ready to stand up to her cancer. When asked where her new-found energy came from, she replied, "I spent the week with my grandkids. It was the first time in months that I was able to really connect with them. Their energy and enthusiasm is contagious, and has given me the second wind I had been looking for to keep on fighting."

The moral of the story: Sometimes the will to fight is more important than the actual battle itself, and sometimes all it takes is a little break to find your will.

As oncologists, we enthusiastically support the idea of chemotherapy holidays for patients receiving chemotherapy for the intent of palliation. Chemotherapy holidays are a break—a holiday—from the monotony of the chemotherapy existence. The obvious worry for most patients is that while taking a break from chemotherapy, their cancer will come back with some type of vengeance. They are worried that if they do not stay on top of the cancer, they will have a worse prognosis and a shorter lifespan. Many times the opposite is actually true. Their longevity may not differ, but their quality of life is improved because their infusions, clinic visits, hospitalizations, and medications do not prevent them from living life to the fullest. Chemotherapy holidays allow patients (and their families) to take some period of time off from chemotherapy (typically weeks or months), and are typically offered to patients who have been receiving chemotherapy for a lengthy period of time. Only your doctor can tell you if a chemotherapy holiday is appropriate for you, so please check with your doctor before deciding to take your own "holiday."

When is the best time to take a break? How long should the rest be? A quarter rest, half rest, whole rest, or more? Together, you and your doctor will need to decide the pace of therapy and where to schedule breaks. The "space between" affords shelter and respite both in music and in life. Rests are vital to your care. Seize and embrace your space between the notes.

CHAPTER 14

Keeping Time

John T. Soper, MD and Nimesh P. Nagarsheth, MD

Pete Seeger, the iconic American folksinger, wrote a song about different purposes to different phases (times) in life. "Turn! Turn! Turn! (to Everything There is a Season)" was originally recorded by him in the early 1960s, but became widely popularized by a version released by the Byrds in 1965 that became a number one pop hit. The lyrics, with the exception of a single concluding line, are essentially a direct quotation from the King James version of the *Bible*, Ecclesiastes 3.1:

1. To every thing there is a season, and a time to every purpose under the heaven;
2. A time to be born, and a time to die; a time to plant, and a time to pluck up that which is planted;
3. A time to kill, and a time to heal; a time to break down, and a time to build up;
4. A time to weep, and a time to laugh; a time to mourn, and a time to dance;
5. A time to cast away stones, and a time to gather stones together; a time to embrace, and a time to refrain from embracing;
6. A time to get, and a time to lose; a time to keep, and a time to cast away;
7. A time to rend, and a time to sow; a time to keep silence, and a time to speak;
8. A time to love, and a time to hate; a time of war, and a time of peace.

Seeger's emphasis was that it was a time for peace, but the original biblical verse generalizes a time to almost all aspects of life.

My co-author, Dr. John Soper, and I have observed that one of the most common questions a patient will ask his or her doctor when initially learning of a diagnosis of cancer is, "How much time do I have left to live?" For most patients, this question has no easy answer. From a physician's perspective, every patient is different, and every cancer is different. This makes it virtually impossible to predict how an individual will respond to a specific treatment plan. Doctors are not fortune tellers and are certainly not gods, so any answer they provide is just an educated guess. What's more, many physicians would not feel comfortable answering the question even if they could, because this is an uncomfortable topic to discuss in general. Still, patients desiring to have an idea of how much time they have left will often ask for at least a time frame, and in many instances this is a reasonable request especially if the patient is motivated to begin planning end-of-life care.

Not surprisingly, doctors generally find talking about the end-of-life inherently difficult. Physicians, after all, spend their careers trying to save lives. But, end-of-life care is an important consideration for everyone regardless of age or current health status, and avoiding the topic can actually be more harmful to the patient and patient's family than having a frank discussion on the topic. Even more importantly, anything can happen in life, and any one of us could suffer an abrupt decline in health due to an accident or other tragedy. This is not meant to depress you, but is a fact of life.

Patients with cancer or other life-threatening illnesses have an identifiable threat that emphasizes the finite duration of the human lifespan; the rest of us only occasionally experience that personal wake-up call. For example, in January 2009, we witnessed the "Miracle on the Hudson" when a passenger plane with 155 people on board was crippled by the loss of engine power and the pilot successfully performed an emergency water landing on the Hudson River. Although there were no fatalities or major injuries from this plane crash, the event was a wake-up call for all those involved (and all those watching) about how delicate life truly is. So no matter who you are or what state of health you may be in, if you haven't thought about end-of-life care, it's about time.

Time

Time is an interesting concept, and means different things to different people. Similar to the many ways one can interpret the meaning of a glass of water filled half way (being half empty versus half full versus just right), a musician's view of time can bring a fresh new perspective to how you view your time on earth and end-of-life care. So, let's take a moment to understand the scientific and artistic aspects of time from a musical point of view. Time is both a science and an art, and arguably nobody understands this concept better than the musician.

Chapter 2 described the scientific basis of music as it applies to musical tones as described by the Greek philosopher Pythagoras. But the scientific mathematical exactness of music also applies to the temporal relationship of notes and rests. In other words, *music occupies space in time in an exacting fashion.* You may think that this concept is obvious, but measuring time in music is not necessarily the same as measuring time in life (otherwise known as *terrestrial time*). For example, knowing that a song that is 3 minutes long tells us nothing about the tempo of the song. In fact, a song that is 5 minutes long could have a much faster tempo or speed than a 3 minute song, or vice versa. What's more, two different songs lasting for 3 minutes each could have the same tempo but have a totally different feeling of time simply because of where the emphasis of each beat is placed.

So, timing in life (as measured by the clock or calendar) only tells us part of the story when it comes to music. Early on, it was realized that music would require its own time terminology in order to properly communicate and coordinate musical ideas and thoughts. Musicians therefore created their own definitions of time measurement, which uses terrestrial time only as a reference.

Specifically, in music the tempo or speed is measured in terms of the number of beats per minute (abbreviated bpm). Each piece of music is divided into groups of beats or measures. The number of beats and emphasis of the beats in each measure are determined by the time signature, which can be the same for the entire piece of music or can change from measure to measure. Time signatures are typically written as a fraction where the top number represents the number of beats in a measure, and the bottom number indicates which type of note value represents one beat. Frequently used time signatures are 4/4 and 2/4 (used in most popular songs including rock, blues, jazz, hip-hop, rap, marches, and dances), 3/4 (waltz time), and 6/8 or 12/8 (swing, blues, rock, jazz, and waltz).

What's truly remarkable about musical timing is that in all its sophistication, it is even more exacting and precise than the terrestrial timing. Now you may say this is impossible! After all, if timing in music is measured relative to the terrestrial minute, then how could it be more precise than terrestrial time itself? The answer may be closer than you think. Maybe even just outside your front door.

For the past 6 years I have lived in an apartment located on Union Square in Manhattan. Just outside my front door is a wall sculpture entitled "Metronome" that is located on the south side of the square. The sculpture is composed of multiple parts including a digital clock and circular structure that expels bursts of steam. Now somewhere in your life experience you have probably seen digital clocks that keep precise time right down to the millisecond, but what makes this clock different is that it is composed of 15 numbers and actually keeps time both forwards and backwards. The first half of the clock tells you the current military time (how much time has passed since midnight), while the second half reads backwards (right to left) and tells you how much time is left in the day. The "Metronome" sculpture attracts the attention of tourists and interested onlookers everyday passing through Union Square, and it is always entertaining to hear the newcomers debate with each other as to what the numbers on the sculpture represent. My favorite tourist response (which seems to be even more popular since the recession has hit) is that the rapidly changing numbers must be the running tally of the national debt. Interestingly, people actually seem relieved when they finally realize the numbers are just part of a fancy clock. But to be accurate, it's not just any clock, it's the "Metronome."

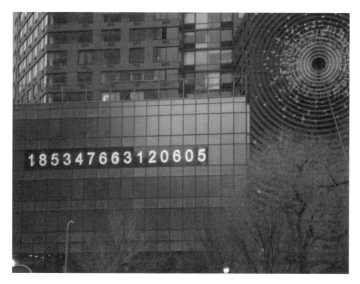

Figure 14-1. Metronome, 1999 by Kristin Jones and Andrew Ginzel. The sculpture is a gift to New York City and is located on the south side of Union Square. Picture by Nimesh P. Nagarsheth, MD.

What's a metronome? A *metronome* is a device used by musicians to mark time. It serves as the musician's "clock" and keeps time in the beat per minute (bpm) format, which can be different for each musical piece, or even different within a piece. There are many different kinds of metronomes, all of which are designed to keep time in various ways. The two more popular kinds include the traditional metronome that has a swinging arm that moves back and forth to mark the beat (this device is often found sitting on top of pianos), and the newer digital metronomes complete with lights and sounds to alert the musician as to the exact location of the beat in relationship to the temporal spatial field of the music. Many digital metronomes can also emphasize the beats in various time signatures.

Musicians have an interesting love/hate relationship with the metronome. It can be your best friend if you feel comfortable with the concept of time, or it can be your worst enemy if you have trouble keeping time. In a band, the percussionist holds the coveted title of the master timekeeper and must be comfortable with this responsibility. Any breech in the percussionist's commitment to keeping time could result in inappropriate speeding up, slowing down, or missed beats. These errors in time keeping can throw off other players in the band, and can result in disastrous consequences for the song. Or simply stated in musician's terms, "It ain't tight."

In order to keep accurate time in the studio (typically when recording), most serious musicians lay down their parts using the guidance of a metronome "click track" to mark the beat while recording. While audible to the musician during the process of recording his or her part, the background click track is almost never heard in the final product. The click track serves as the time marker for all the members in the band to assure everyone is playing in synchrony. Believe it or not, playing along with a click track can be one of the most harrowing experiences a musician can face.

Even the most talented and experienced musicians can be reduced to the feeling of an amateur when stepping into the studio if they are not accustomed to playing with a click track behind them. This is because most musicians, whether they realize it or not, have a tendency to either speed up or slow down when playing live. In music, the metronome is considered the great equalizer and fortunately (or unfortunately for some), the metronome never lies. If the musician is not playing in time, the metronome will uncover this lack of precision and the musician will be immediately made aware of his or her error.

But with all this talk about the precision of musical timing, I still need to somehow convince you that the musician's time is even more accurate than the time we keep in real life. Although the metronome provides the foundation for my argument, this is going to be tougher than I thought. In situations like this, a little champaign and celebration can go a long way to help brighten the mood. So before we move on, let's break out a bottle of your finest bubbly and take a second to remember our New Year's Eve celebration count down in 2008. Believe it or not, your celebration highlights the minor inconsistency of time keeping here on earth.

For those of you who did not notice (or maybe already have forgotten), on New Years Eve of 2008, the timekeepers of the world delayed the beginning of the year 2009 by 1 second. So, people counting down to 2009 actually had to count 1 extra second before the New Year officially started. An extra second inserted in this manner has been referred to as a *leap second* (akin to the leap years we add to our calendar every 4 years) and actually occurs more often than most people realize (from 1972 to 2009 we added 24 leap seconds to our clocks and watches). The introduction of the leap second has been mandated by the world's experts in time keeping in order to remedy the discrepancies between two very different ways of keeping time in real life. The original way of keeping time, based on astronomical calculations and the earth's rotation speed, has been slowing down because the earth's rotation continues to slow down a rate of about two-thousandths of a second per day. A more precise method of time keeping using atomic clocks (accurate up to one-billionth of a second per day) is based on the nuclear physics of cesium atoms and has been in use since the 1950s. Therefore, in order to accommodate the difference in timing between the more precise atomic clocks and the ever-slowing time as measured by the earth's rotation, two methods are utilized; a leap second is periodically added to terrestrial time, and the atomic clocks are stopped for 1 second every 500 days or so. By employing these two corrective measures, we are able to reset the clock so to speak until the time when another second needs to be added. Thus, although musical timing never requires adjustment to make up for the naturally slowing rotation of the earth, terrestrial timing requires constant adjustments to remain accurate.

With all that said about the strict sense of timing in music, I will tell you that musicians are the first to recognize the artistry behind keeping time. Musicians will often use terminology such as *playing in the groove* or *rocking the beat*, which serves to add some artistic interpretation to the otherwise straightforward beat. Specifically, if you were to hear a song with a beat that was 100% on line with the click track, it would be so exact that there would be no human touch to the beat, and it would likely sound like a sterile computer-generated piece of music. Although very precise and accurate, a beat this straight and exact might make it extremely difficult for the listener to feel connected with the song. To remedy this problem, musicians typically like to play "in the groove." The groove is not a physical place, but a feeling. In general, each song has its own characteristic grooves, and different musicians will find different grooves for the same piece of music. Finding the groove is an art (not a science) and typically involves intentionally playing slightly ahead of the beat (*pushing the beat*), tightly on the beat (*burying the beat*), or playing behind the beat (*laying back on the beat*). These playing styles are the musician's subtle interpretations of keeping time, and when performed intentionally can add life to an otherwise monotonous beat. By balancing the science of timing and the art of playing in the groove, musicians are able to remain precise and still connect with their audience at the same time.

There are many ways to find your groove in life between the opening count and the final chord. Similar to how a musician can play behind the beat, on the beat, or in front of the beat, you can view time from the past, present, or future. Each of these viewpoints offers advantages and disadvantages, and each serves a particular purpose during different times in our lives. At any given time, any one or all of these ways of looking at time might be in play. Learning how to balance these perspectives on time is the key to being comfortable with end-of-life care.

Based on the above discussion, it is clear that musicians have a unique perspective when it comes to matters of time, for in music time is all encompassing. As an organic, evolving process during a performance, good musicians are constantly listening to their bandmates and making subtle adjustments to their time keeping so that all elements of the music are in concordance. Musicians realize that once a song has started, there is no way to stop the clock or go backwards in a song, and any attempt we make to do so simply squanders precious time (a lesson taken from Chapter 9). In music, just as in life, time continuously passes. The logical conclusion therefore must be to live life to its fullest and play your song to the best of your ability. Of course, I realize that this is easier said than done, and that life is full of twists and turns with many unexpected challenges and set backs. Although there is no way to go back in time, simply looking at time from a different viewpoint could add new perspectives to your life (the glass is half full).

When N.E.D. began assembling original songs during the summer of 2008, I came across lyrics that dealt with the passage of time written by Doctors John Soper and John Boggess (partners in the Division of Gynecologic Oncology at the University of North Carolina, Chapel Hill). I was struck by the incredible insight these lyrics provided me regarding the passage of time and positive thoughts on end-of-life issues. From a unique background as an accomplished musician coupled with his years of experience caring for cancer patients, Dr. Soper is a true expert on issues of time. In the remaining part of this chapter, Dr. Soper generously shares his inspiration and thoughts behind the creation of the song "Waiting on Time," and discusses his insights on time as it relates to end-of-life care.

In the Words of Dr. John Soper

I had originally written the lyrics for "Waiting on Time" from the perspective of a patient's husband who was waiting with his wife in a physician's office for a discussion of end-of-life issues. The minutes seem to drag by and he reflects back on their life together (Example 1, original first verse).

Example 1

Waiting on Time (original first verse)

© 2009 by N.E.D.

Lyrics by John T. Soper and John F. Boggess

Music by John T. Soper

(*Verse 1*)
Waiting in the room with the clock up on the wall
Distant voices, distant footsteps echo down the hall
And the man in the corner with his wife
Stares away down the hallways of his life
Cause they'd always be together
And make it through this time
But for all their prayers and promises
They reached the end of the line

Altogether this was a very dark set of lyrics and somewhat depressing. In the process of rewriting the song, we increased the tempo slightly and changed the focus of the lyrics, while keeping the same chord structure and basic melody. In the re-write, the protagonist is nearing the end of his life in a metaphorical railway station, waiting for the inevitable and remembering his past life with his deceased wife (Example 2, re-write full lyrics).

Example 2

Waiting on Time (re-write full lyrics)

© 2009 by N.E.D.
Lyrics by John T. Soper and John F. Boggess
Music by John T. Soper

(*Verse 1/Chorus*)
Waiting on time at the station, the whistle blows
My eyes are fixed upon the door
Eighty-two years since this journey first began
Eighty-two years since I was born
And as I fumble with the ticket in my hand
You cast a shadow from the door

Your radiant beauty
So soft and soothing
And I am suddenly transported

(*Verse 2/Chorus*)
To a time when we first lay together
A different year a different place
We always knew we'd be together, you and I
I saw my future in your face
But it's been so many years since you and I walked the line
And as the whistle blows, I'm running out of time
So I gaze

At your radiant beauty
So soft and soothing
And I am suddenly transported

(*Verse 3/Chorus*)
Among the years we stumbled you and I
Separated by the passage of time
And when your star fell from the heavens, I lost my way
Without your light to be my guide
So now that I see you in the doorway to my journey's end
Take my hand and I'll step inside

Such radiant beauty
So soft and soothing
We'll live forever on the other side

By virtue of these changes, the song became a much more uplifting and positive song, even though still dealing with many of the same themes as the original song. Getting closer to the end-of-life does not have to be a depressing experience, but can actually be a celebrated experience.

Time is an interesting concept, and has different definitions for different people. At its basic meaning, time is a system used to place events in sequence (distant past, recent past, a moment ago, near future, or distant future), to compare the durations of events or the intervals between them, and to quantify the motions of objects. Of interest, because it takes a fraction of a second for the brain to process sensory information, it could be said that we are all actually "living in the past," rather than experiencing the present. Time is usually divided by measuring repetitive events: before clocks were invented, a day was measured from sunrise to sunrise, a month by the changing phases of the moon, and a year was based on the revolution of the earth around the sun as realized by the natural changing seasons and the organization of constellations. The earliest clocks used energy from gravity, a spring, or a swinging pendulum to measure time. The development of accurate standardized chronometers was essential for navigation. Current atomic clocks, as discussed above, are based on measuring the energy released by repetitive changes in energy states among cesium atoms and are accurate to miniscule fractions of a second!

> Interestingly, the word *time* is often used as a synecdoche. "Time the runner" (rather than "measure the length of time the runner ran the distance"), "doing time" (instead of "spending a length of time in prison"), "time heals all wounds" (rather than "passage of time promotes healing"), and "time out" (rather than "I need to take some length of time away from this activity") are all very familiar examples.

On a much deeper level, time is the basis for many religious and philosophical treatises. In this context, time is often thought of as a fourth dimension, and is often viewed as a subjective rather than an objective interval. To the latter point, many of us are aware of the impression that time passes more quickly as we age, possibly reflecting our perception that the passage of time is related to the total amount of time that we have experienced previously. In addition to the above, certain states of awareness may change our perception of time. For example, many athletes report a sensation of time slowing down when they are concentrating on a task such as hitting a baseball, where the pitched ball seems to float toward them in slow motion. Cancer patients often relate the agonizingly slow passage of time they experience while waiting for crucial test results or procedures (similar to Example 1).

Understanding music adds a whole new perspective to the meaning of time. For example, in music, one aspect of time keeping is the feel of the beat throughout a musical piece. Another example involves synchronizing the beginning and ending of a musical performance. Because it is crucial that all members of a musical group are coordinated in their understanding of the tempo and beat, most groups designate one member of the band to provide a "count in" to indicate the tempo and time signature of the piece. This is often provided by the drummer or percussionist. However, the conductor, lead vocalist, or the instrumentalist who opens a tune with a solo may be the band member who provides the "count in." Laurence Welk was famous for his "a-one and-a-two" count in that he used to kick off countless tunes on his television show, but the count in may be communicated in nonverbal forms as well. On most recordings, the count in is not heard, but the band starts together. One familiar and effective opening to a song is the distinctive chord that starts the Beatles' "Hard Day's Night." This was pieced together in the studio with guitars, bass, and piano, and is followed by a silent count in before the song begins. Whether loud or silent, the count provides the structure needed to keep the group together. In music as in life, time is your friend.

Doctors are constantly focusing on new and innovative ways to increase the survival times of cancer patients, which often involves treatment plans using radical surgery, aggressive chemotherapy, and/or significant radiation therapy. But the benefit of added time must always be weighed against the risks of the treatment toxicities. Thus, before formulating a treatment plan, the doctor and patient must discuss the goals of treatment. This includes the likelihood of cure (or long-term remission) with each treatment option, as well as the incremental benefit to adding additional forms of treatment along with their associated side effects. While many patients will want to "do everything," it is probably not advisable to add a treatment that has a 5% chance of serious side-effects if the original therapy has an excellent probability of producing a cure on its own. While focusing on survival time is important, doctors (and their patients) must not lose sight of the fact that maintaining a good quality of life is a key part of the equation. In fact, many would argue that time without quality of life is worse than not having that time at all.

Perhaps the most challenging decision-making scenario for physicians, patients, and their families is in situations where the chance for cure is very low and the focus of care is shifted to palliating, relieving, or postponing the effects of cancer. In this case, we are no longer trying to increase survival time, but rather improve the quality of life of the patient during the time she has left. Most often, this occurs when there is recurrence of disease after potentially curative treatments have already been given, or there is progression of the cancer during treatment. I believe that it is incumbent on the physician to have a frank discussion with the patient and as many family members as possible (and allowed by the patient) about the reality of the situation. All options for management should be discussed, including the fact that comfort care is part of the treatment strategy if we are not successful in controlling the disease, or the patient cannot tolerate treatment side effects.

In times like these, I emphasize the need for the patient to think through her wishes in regard to extremes of medical care: Would she wish to be placed on a ventilator, undergo dialysis, or invasive major surgery? I discuss the formulation of a living will, assigning medical power of attorney if she cannot make decisions in the future, and discuss the importance of communicating her wishes to all of her family members. This foreshadowing at a time before entering the final phases of a life-threatening disease is extremely helpful in future discussions, especially when there are no other reasonable options for active treatment with surgery, radiation therapy, chemotherapy, or other potential agents. All too often, physicians have to deal with patients who have not communicated their desires to family, are unable to communicate their wishes because of medical circumstances, and have family members who cannot agree on the patient's care. It is important for physicians to communicate that even when no active treatment is available for her cancer, he or she will still be involved in the patient's care. This holds true especially for the palliation of the effects of cancer, such as pain control, bowel obstruction, and other potential complex issues.

Several years ago, I treated a young woman with a rare and aggressive form of uterine sarcoma. Initially diagnosed at the time of a hysterectomy, she was treated with chemotherapy, and after a remission of several years' duration the sarcoma recurred in the upper abdomen. There was no evidence of other sites of disease, so we performed a radical tumor debulking surgery. Despite further treatment, the cancer recurred again, but this time it extensively involved the liver. Her chances of cure or even response to chemotherapy were very small, so I had a long discussion with the patient and her husband about the goals of treatment at that phase of her disease. We decided to try chemotherapy again in an attempt to palliate her symptoms, but agreed we would stop the treatment if there was not any evidence of response after a few treatments or if she developed severe side effects from the chemotherapy. She was fortunate to have a significant response to treatment with very little toxicity. During this time, she traveled extensively, was able to remain physically active, and finished writing a textbook. After 18 months, however, the cancer recurred yet again and did not respond to chemotherapy. At that point in time, we did not have any reasonable chance of response to additional chemotherapy, and she was physically unable to tolerate additional treatment.

After our discussion about transitioning into end-of-life care, I said something to the effect that I wished I could have been more successful in treating her disease. She drew herself up, looked resolutely at me, and said: "But Dr. Soper, I do consider myself one of your successes." She noted her palliative treatments gave her the ability to maximize what time she had left. She had the opportunity to discuss her situation with her daughters and husband, had written her will, had assigned medical power of attorney to her husband, and had emotionally prepared herself for this phase of her life. She was able to die peacefully at home, surrounded by her family, with minimal pain thanks to home hospice nursing care.

In the United States, discussions about death and the process of dying have been often pushed into the shadows, as if death is not part of the living process. Fortunately, there appears to be a gradually changing attitude toward this subject, with more open discussions of end-of-life issues in the lay press. It is time to discuss these topics more candidly, hopefully providing you with information and food for thought. I will reference several web sites that contain relevant information. To begin with, the American Association of Retired Persons (www.aarp.org/families) has information on a variety of these issues with links to other resources, including information about wills, caregiving, and financial planning.

When patients are admitted to a hospital, unless there is documentation noting otherwise, physicians are legally and ethically bound to try all reasonable means to prolong life even if a patient cannot express his or her wishes. The documentation regarding patient wishes can take on many related forms.

An *Advanced Directive* is a statement of the types of care that you would or would not wish to have under different situations and is signed in front of a witness. This could include avoiding mechanical ventilation, dialysis, tube or intravenous feedings, or major surgery if you were not able to make decisions and had a major irreversible fatal illness or were in an irreversible coma. These are most often prepared as part of the process during an elective admission to a hospital and become part of the medical record. Different states have different laws governing the limitations of an advanced directive. Most require a notarized and witnessed signature with the witnesses stating that you understand the decisions, are of sound mind, and are competent to make decisions.

Similar to an advanced directive, a *Living Will* is a legal document that specifies treatments that you would wish to have if faced with a life-threatening or terminal illness. The National Institute of Medicine and National Institutes of Health have brief descriptions with informative links to other sites that can provide guidance in preparing these documents (www.nlm.nih.gov/medlineplus/advancedirectives.html), and several of these sites offer state-specific forms for advanced directives and living wills, such as the National Hospice and Palliative Care Organization (www.caringinfo.org).

A *Do Not Resuscitate (DNR)* order is another type of advanced directive that takes the form of an order placed in the hospital chart by your physician. It requires that physicians document having a discussion with you (or your healthcare proxy) about your disease, its prognosis, options for management, and that you do not wish to undergo cardiopulmonary resuscitation (CPR) if a respiratory or cardiac arrest occurs. If a DNR order is entered into the chart during an admission, all physicians and nurses caring for the patient will be aware of this designation and will not subject the patient to invasive attempts to prolong life in the event of an acute arrest.

Importantly, having a legally specified person who will act as your healthcare proxy or durable power of attorney is binding in all states. This person is selected by you to make medical decisions on your behalf if you are incapacitated. Most often a spouse or other family member is selected for this role, but trusted friends are often recruited if family members are not available or live far away. In some families, feelings can be hurt (or arguments can ensue) if one of several children is selected as the healthcare power of attorney. This can often be avoided by having a frank discussion with all family members regarding the reasons for selection of the person for this position. Some patients will document one (or more) alternative person to exercise medical power of attorney. It is also important to discuss thoroughly your preferences for care issues to determine that the designated healthcare proxy is comfortable with this responsibility and will act on your behalf, according to your wishes rather than his or her philosophy.

The line between palliative care and hospice care is blurred, and often defined rather arbitrarily in terms of time. The concept of palliative care is centered on an emphasis for relieving pain, suffering, or other effects caused by a disease rather than trying to cure or treat the underlying disease. In reality, all medical care should be palliative, even during self-limited diseases, because physicians should always try to reduce the physical and emotional toll of an illness. In hospice care, the focus is on providing palliative care during the final phases of a terminal disease. In most instances this requires the physician to state that the patient is expected to live less than 6 months and have little chance of significant benefit from additional disease-specific forms of treatment (such as surgery, chemotherapy, or radiation). The phrases *terminal cancer, less than 6 months' life expectancy*, and *no benefit from further treatment* can be very intimidating for the patient and family. They often wrongly believe that their physician has "given up" on providing care.

Because these are emotionally loaded terms, I choose to introduce hospice care as part of the treatment options early on in discussions of treatment strategies for advanced or recurrent cancers, as mentioned previously. I usually preface this discussion with the question: "Why do we treat cancer, anyway?" The obvious answer is that we treat cancer to try to limit the effects of cancer and the effects of treatment on the quality of a patient's life. In situations where there are no good treatment options, or the patient is unable to tolerate treatment, palliative care is required. I always ask that my patients honestly communicate to me when they do not believe that they can physically or emotionally endure more treatment. In return, I promise them that I will always be honest regarding the risks and benefits of treatment, and will inform them when we are at a time in their disease when further treatment is not likely to provide a benefit. I revisit this discussion any time we re-initiate or consider changing treatment.

Hospice care usually provides home-based services for daily, often prolonged, assessments and interventions by nurses or other trained health professionals. Many hospices are commercial home nursing businesses, although some hospice services are entirely organized and run by volunteers as a non-profit organization. Medicare has special reimbursement and funding for patients placed in hospice care that allows this extra home care, without having to pay more out-of-pocket for home nursing care above and beyond what is covered for patients who are not in hospice care. In addition to providing home-based services, hospice units in several larger communities will have inpatient facilities to provide care for terminal patients who cannot be cared for in their homes. The American Hospice Foundation (http://www.americanhospice.org/index.php), the Hospice Foundation (http://www.hospicefoundation.org/), Hospice Patients Alliance (http://www.hospicepatients.org/), and the National Hospice and Palliative Care Organization (http://www.caringinfo.org) provide valuable online resources for patients and families considering hospice care.

Before beginning home hospice care, it is important to ensure that the patient and all family members who will be providing care are ready for this transition in the medical status of the patient. A survey is made of the patient's home to determine whether special equipment, such as an adjustable hospital bed or bedside commode, is needed. The availability and ability of family members to provide care and administer medications is assessed. The hospice patient is visited in her home environment early on to determine the amount of daily nursing care and level of interventions that are needed.

Many misconceptions exist about hospice care. Some patients and their family members believe that accepting hospice care means that basic medical treatments for medical conditions such as infections are not allowed, that they cannot be admitted to a hospital for care when they have accepted outpatient hospice services, or that patients must be bed-bound before they can be cared for in a hospice setting. On the contrary, hospice patients are able to be treated with non-invasive interventions that will improve their quality of life. Examples of these may include transfusions for anemia, antibiotics for infections, and adjusting medications used to treat heart failure. Under certain circumstances, palliative radiation treatments, chemotherapy, and minor surgical procedures are appropriate and allowed.

For example, appropriate surgical procedures include drainage of fluid accumulation in the abdomen (ascites) or chest (pleural effusion) caused by cancer.

Inpatient hospital admission is used when the medical situation has deteriorated because of an acute, self-limited condition that cannot be managed in the outpatient setting but might be reversed with appropriate care. Specific situations might include hospitalization for intravenous antibiotics to control a complicated infection of the kidneys (pyelonephritis) or lungs (pneumonia), starting blood thinners to treat a blood clot, or for acute treatment and stabilization of a bowel obstruction. In the majority of these admissions, the goal is to improve the patient's condition so that returning to the home environment is possible.

I actively encourage patients to consider hospice care, if possible, before they become bed-bound or have an expected survival of only a few weeks. This allows the patient and the family the opportunity to adjust to the hospice care environment and emphasis before they require intense daily care. The patients are able to meet the hospice caregivers before they are mentally clouded by medications or disease and can accept them as partners in their health care as they make the transition into a medical state that usually requires more care as their disease progresses. In contrast, I have witnessed some very awkward transitions into hospice care—delayed until it was obvious that death was very near. In those instances, the patient required complicated arrangements for home care, the family members were not prepared for their active participation in the home care, or the family had unrealistic expectations about home hospice care. Furthermore, the hospice agency often had to scramble in these situations to provide high-intensity care with minimal preparation. Clearly, this is not ideal.

In many cancer patients the disease process interrupts eating, drinking, or metabolism of nutrients. In some patients, the cancer mechanically produces a partial or complete bowel blockage caused by spread to the intestines or accumulation of fluid in the abdomen (ascites). Sometimes the side effects of treatment such as radiation therapy to the head and neck, esophagus, or intestines may directly interfere with eating. Furthermore, weight loss and muscle wasting are frequently seen late in the course of an advanced malignancy, caused by diversion of nutrients to the cancer rather than to normal tissues or caused by nonspecific loss of appetite. It is tempting to use intravenous total parenteral nutrition (TPN) or tube feedings to attempt to maintain nutrition. I usually discourage these forms of feedings in hospice patients because it is rare that these provide any long-term benefit. In some situations, the feedings will only prolong life for a short interval of time when the patient may be battling with control of severe pain or other symptoms of terminal cancer. In patients who have little pain, intravenous (IV) fluids may help them retain mental clarity so that they can interact with family members for a short time longer.

My goal in providing care to my cancer patients is to try to sense the pulse of their interaction with their disease. By maintaining this sensitivity throughout my interactions, I hope that I can time appropriate interventions so that the cancer is controlled and that a high quality of life is maintained throughout. Increasing survival times while maintaining a good quality of life for my patients is my goal. Often the hardest decisions come near the end of the patient's life, where the balance must be shifted if possible to provide the patient with the means and support for a peaceful, dignified, and pain-free death in the place of their choosing. For most patients death at home surrounded by family would be ideal. Hospice and other available support services provide the means for many patients to achieve that goal.

PART V

Hope and the Future

CHAPTER 15

The Show Must Go On

William "Rusty" Robinson, MD and Nimesh P. Nagarsheth, MD

Long before the creation of N.E.D., I (Dr. Nagarsheth) had joined a Beatles and Rolling Stones cover band called Come Together. Prior to my joining Come Together, the band had already been well-established in the New York City music scene and played gigs on a regular basis (usually one gig every couple of months or so). The musicians in this band all had professional day jobs (and good ones at that), so rehearsals and the periodic gigs were manageable and actually fit in well with everyone's busy schedules. But after a series of communication breakdowns, personality conflicts, and general lack of "satisfaction" with their drummer, the group kicked him out of the band and opened up a search for his replacement.

> Just as an aside, this brings up an interesting point for those of you who are unfamiliar with the inner workings of rock bands. For some unknown reason that I am still trying to understand, most rock bands have a hard time staying together for any lengthy period of time. Now this is just my observation, and I have seen no statistics to back this up (and am not sure if any statistics actually exist on this topic). But if you have ever watched a documentary of a band on MTV or VH1, I am willing to bet there was some discussion about conflict and strife and maybe even a change of personnel in the group, or even a complete disintegration of the group. Just like any relationship (including marriages for that matter), those that make it through the rough patches are likely the ones who have been grounded with healthy communication skills, laughter, and fun.

As circumstance would have it, living down the hall from Come Together's bass player (a Wall Street executive at the time), I was invited to audition for the open position of drummer. In all honesty, I was initially hesitant to take on another commitment in my life, given the already busy hospital hours I held. However, persuaded by the Wall Street tactics unleashed on me, I did eventually audition for the band, and was formally invited to join the band a few days later.

After playing regularly for about a year, Come Together took on a life of its own. With enough repetition and practice, each of us had now mastered our parts, and the band was able to take the show to the next level and began functioning like a well-oiled machine. And just like an engine that requires many parts to run smoothly, this machine required each of us to be on top of our game, every gig. In the music industry, many refer to this Nirvana-like state as *being in the zone*. With each gig, our chemistry strengthened and our energy was contagious. The crowds grew and the enthusiasm for the band spread quickly. Although we realized that each member of the band was essential, what we didn't realize is that this also meant we were somewhat dependent on each other. What would happen to our well-oiled machine if one of the band members became ill or for some other reason couldn't make a gig? We would soon learn the answer to this question (the hard way).

During one of our 2006 rehearsals, our lead singer brought up a potential gig opportunity for the band in Las Vegas at the lavish Wynn Resort. A year before, we had been flown to Las Vegas and played a similar gig at the hottest club in the Wynn Resort and had a blast. Living the dreams of rock stars, we booked this show and began planning the set list. However, this gig was going to be a tough one to pull off as it required at least 2 full days off from our New York City jobs during a busy time of year. It seemed our music career finally reached the breaking point of impinging on our day jobs. Still, where there is a will, there is a way, and we were going to make our best effort to work through our individual scheduling conflicts.

We reached Las Vegas piecemeal, all on separate flights based on our schedules and availability. By the afternoon of the gig, all of us had made it safely to the desert except for our lead guitarist. I vividly remember walking in front of the water fountains at the Bellagio asking the rest of the group if anyone had heard from him. And just then the phone rang; Joe was stuck at Newark Liberty International Airport with a flight delay. We did the math, even if he somehow miraculously made his flight at this point, he would not make the gig in time. We were on our own. For the first time ever in our years of playing together as a band, we would have to play without a key piece of the machine we had built. With no preparation for this unfortunate turn of events, we were dejected and felt the chemistry bleeding from our engine. But, then those magic words were uttered by our ever persuasive and optimistic Wall Street bassist, "The show must go on!" And right he was. We had no choice but to make this work. We owed it to our fans, to the Wynn Resort, and most importantly to ourselves. We just needed to believe in ourselves and we could pull this off.

The show did go on, and the band rose to the occasion. Of course, the show was not the same without Joe, but it was special in its own way. The crowd did not seem to notice our short-handedness (or if they did, they were kind enough not to tell us), and we discovered our six-cylinder engine could function well with only five cylinders during emergencies. In addition, we realized the importance of teamwork and how to deal with an unexpected situation. Much more, we learned that anything can happen in a live performance, just as anything can happen in life. So while it is good to have a group (or family) whose members depend on each other, the individuals in the group need to be able to adapt to the unexpected and function somewhat independently as well.

The fact that the show must go on does not just refer to music and performance, but is a lesson for life with cancer. Life doesn't stop because you have cancer. Your show must go on, and you need to find at least a temporary role for the bad actor of cancer in your life production. Just as in the performing arts, there are ways to prepare for the unexpected.

Preparing for the unexpected is far better than scrambling and making haphazard adjustments at the last minute. Looking back on our nerve racking experience of having to put on a show without one of our key players, we could have done many things differently to prepare for Joe's absence. First, we could have paid more attention to the times of the flights and even performed some research as to how often flights are delayed from Newark (in my experience—they are always delayed). A simple look at the weather report could have also given us an idea of potential flight delays. Second, we could have used a small portion of our many hours of rehearsal time to prepare for the scenario of how to proceed if we are missing a member of the group. Simple exercises such as hearing how a song would sound with only one guitarist, or with the back-up singer taking the lead role, etc., would have given us a much better idea of what we were up against when we got that phone call confirming our worst nightmare, and would have taken away our fear of the unexpected.

Although you may never need to use it, it is always a good idea to have a back-up plan ready in case of the occasional monkey wrench that may be thrown your way. Preparation is key. Your life with cancer may not be the same as your life before cancer, but it can still be a positive experience.

Probably one of the best tools (not to be confused with a defense mechanism) we have readily available to us to handle an unexpected occurrence is humor. When I think of humor in this setting, I am reminded of a holiday musical that my seven-year-old niece recently took part in which was put on by the theater group of a local community college. During a transition between scenes (with the lights out), one of the back stage helpers accidentally tilted a dining room table prop and all of the loose silverware and dishes that had been carefully laid out on top of the table came crashing down on the stage. Without hesitation, the members of the cast quickly joined the clean up efforts and helped to re-construct the prop and, aside from the loud noise and a little commotion, the next scene started without a major hitch (from the actors' point of view). Despite this incredible recovery, the audience initially was not very forgiving. Similar to the curious drivers slowing down to catch a glimpse of the scene of an accident, the audience had been easily distracted as witnessed by the restlessness and low level whispering that persisted well after the lights had been switched on signaling the start of the next scene. Realizing the need to intervene quickly, one of the adult seasoned actors made a brilliant spontaneous move. Instead of pretending that the accident did not occur, he brought it front and center and commented to one of the other actors on stage in a loud and bold voice, "I need to get you a new table that can withstand the earthquakes you have been experiencing here." And with his quick wit combined with his candid acknowledgment of a mishap that had just occurred live on stage, this actor diffused the tense and awkward situation that had been created moments prior and made the audience once again feel at ease. In fact, the spontaneity actually added a human touch to the scripted play and made for an enjoyable and memorable experience.

Laughter is a great medicine that is available to everyone and is free of charge. When faced with difficult situations regarding cancer, remember your show must go on, and humor and laughter have incredible powers that can help get you through this period. Performers and artists use humor to diffuse tense, anxiety-provoking situations, and so can you.

At a recent N.E.D. rehearsal, Dr. William "Rusty" Robinson (bass player) and I began an interesting discussion about the different ways to interpret the phrase "the show must go on" with regard to the cancer patient. For Rusty, these words brought back memories of one of his most engaging and optimistic patients. When he shared her inspiring story with me that day, I knew immediately that her story belonged here. This is an example of one woman's incredible quest to keep her show going despite an unexpected appearance from the bad actor of cancer.

In the Words of Dr. Rusty Robinson

I have occasionally struggled to recollect things that have happened to me in the past. My friends mention a name that I don't recall, and I've found it a little frustrating. I worry that I am forgetting important things that made me who I am.

I've managed to overcome that frustration by actively trying to reflect on the things that have influenced me over the years, rather than simply recall specific events or names. It's a fascinating exercise that I recommend wholeheartedly. One memory begets another, and then another, and so on. Soon, you are reconstructing the various periods of your life in great detail.

I was engaged in one of these mental exercises recently, during a discussion with Dr. Nagarsheth about the meaning of the phrase, "The show must go on." I was reminded about how our local gynecologic cancer survivors' group was started from one person's desire to keep the show going. This group was founded and named "Princess Warriors" almost 10 years ago by a patient of mine I'll refer to as Rhonda.

Rhonda was 34-years-old when she was diagnosed with stage IIIC ovarian cancer. If her life can be described as a "play," as in the words of Shakespeare, then I think she would say everything up until her diagnosis was just setting the stage for the appearance of the antagonist, ovarian cancer. From then on, her life (her play) accelerated into the realm of epic theatre.

Rhonda was undergoing surgery with the intention of performing a hysterectomy for the presumptive diagnosis of endometriosis. In fact, she had widely metastatic ovarian cancer. I performed a standard ovarian cancer operation, removing the visible tumor (referred to as *radical debulking*) along with her ovaries and uterus. Rhonda saw me for the first time later that day.

As I explained what we'd found and what that meant for her, I could see most of the five so-called "stages" of death and dying flash across her face at once. I explained the need for chemotherapy, the side effects that came with the treatment, the surveillance process, and the prognosis associated with advanced ovarian cancer. As she confided to me later, she hated me at that moment, but slowly worked through those feelings over the next few months.

Rhonda came from a blue-collar background, was relatively uneducated, and yet was remarkably insightful. She eventually achieved the emotional maturity that so many people in this world strive for unsuccessfully. She loved her two teenage daughters and her husband deeply, even when they didn't understand what was happening and reacted poorly. And she understood the concept of the phrase, "The show must go on." In fact, her show was just entering its most dramatic scenes.

Princess Warriors was the product of Rhonda's mind and energy at this time. She was looking for emotional support shortly after her diagnosis, and was directed to a breast cancer survivor group in our facility, which is the only female cancer survivor group in the area. This was not a good match for Rhonda's interests. Rhonda perceived that they looked at her as an outsider, with her modest social status and her cancer from below the waist. One meeting was all it took to convince Rhonda that something was missing from the menu of survivor opportunities available.

Rhonda finished her chemotherapy and achieved a complete response, which meant she clinically had no evidence of disease (N.E.D.). She directed her energy at that point into the creation of a survivors group just for gynecologic cancer patients. With the help of one of our nurse practitioners and myself serving as cheerleaders,

Rhonda mobilized a group of like-minded survivors and arranged a series of fund-raising events. They managed to develop a self-supporting program that has now assisted several hundred gynecologic cancer patients with everything from regular support group meetings to paying for expensive prescriptions. They have sponsored a room designated for gynecologic cancer families at the local Ronald McDonald house, and a chair in the donation area of the local blood bank. Perhaps most interesting, the Princess Warriors organization has attracted interest from physicians and nurses from facilities across the United States seeking to establish similar groups.

Rhonda's play ended when she succumbed to her disease after a 4-year long battle that included several surgeries and multiple chemotherapy regimens. Her final scene with me was in a hospice setting, where she thanked me repeatedly for all I had done, despite the fact that she was dying. She understood life and death in a way that few do, and that I hope I can some day.

Princess Warriors was Rhonda's precious child until the end. I believe her greatest tribute outside her family is that the organization has survived her and continues to grow. Princess Warriors is currently working with the Western Association of Gynecologic Oncologists to promote both graduate medical education and public education regarding gynecologic cancers. Rhonda and Princess Warriors have certainly been among the most important influences on me. Reading her story is similar to watching a play, in a sense. It allows the reader to suspend reality briefly and put yourself in her shoes. We can then try to imagine what we would have done in her situation.

Some have defined art as any object, drawing, play, book, film, etc., that attempts to elicit an emotional response from the viewer. Rhonda's story, her play, certainly fits that definition. And yet, it is not a tragedy as she was able to keep the show going to a triumphant conclusion despite adversity. I believe Rhonda would have suggested that the most important part of her life came after she was diagnosed. I challenge cancer patients, or anyone facing adversity, to find inspiration from Rhonda's play. Success in life can only occur so long as we continue to believe *The Show Must Go On*.

We all owe enormous debts of gratitude to those around us. For doctors, it's no different. We learn and grow from patients, from colleagues, from friends, and from family in ways you could never imagine. As long as you do your best and yet recognize the limitations we all have, you must accept what life has in store. The people who can do that, those who truly understand that *The Show Must Go On*, have found one of the true keys to a fulfilling life.

CHAPTER 16

The Live Performance and the Meaning of Cancer

Nimesh P. Nagarsheth, MD

Choosing the Composition, Arrangement, and Details of Your Performance

Now that you have learned about the ins and outs of music, from the ancient origins of percussion to the modern day performance of rock bands (and everything in between), it's time to put your newly acquired artistic knowledge to work. In the world of music, the live performance provides the artist with the opportunity to interact with his or her audience, and it's where a lifetime of practice and hard work culminate. The energy and anticipation leading up to a concert can be both anxiety-provoking and electrifying, and the challenge for the musician is to stay focused during this time, as there are important decisions to be made.

In the process of getting ready, musicians go through a ritual of sorts, which includes choosing the composition, musical arrangement, and details of the show. They call on their experience as well as on the advice of those around them to help guide them through this process to ensure the best outcome. In this chapter, following the model of how musicians prepare for a live performance, you will discover how to live life to the fullest everyday in what I like to refer to as your *life performance* with cancer. Through this artistic approach, you will learn how to call on a lifetime of experiences to make your stand against cancer, and gain a better understanding behind the meaning of life with cancer.

Choosing Your Composition

A musician without a song to play is like a salesperson without a product to sell. The first thing a musician must do when getting ready for a performance is to choose the composition (the song or songs) he or she wishes to play. While the song preferences may be straightforward to the musician, typically several factors will come into play when putting together a *song list* (also known as a *set list*). Most importantly, in order to move the listener, the musician must truly enjoy and believe in the music. Because the musician does not exist in isolation, he or she must also take into consideration input from other members of the band, the record label, and of course the audience, as each one of these groups is intimately connected and contributes to the success of the performance. Finally, the pieces should be appropriate for the musician's talent and skill level, as he or she needs to play these songs with confidence in a live performance setting.

> On the popular television show "American Idol," just before voting a singer off the show, the judges will often say something to the effect, "You're a good singer, but the song you chose was not the right song for your voice or personality." For a musician, choosing the song that best suits his or her talent is critical, and can make the difference between making the cut or getting cut.

In the context of your performance, your "song" represents your disposition, or your outlook if you will, on life with cancer. It touches on all aspects of your life including how cancer affects your career, family, values, who you want to be, and how you want others to view you. Your song can be fun or serious, loud (*forte*) or soft (*piano*), etc., and reflects how comfortable you are in your own skin (believing in your song). Your support from family and friends (gathering input from your "band"), your bond with caregivers and medical team (possessing a strong rapport with your "record label"), and your relationship with community and society (connecting with your "audience") are all part of the equation. Your song thus encompasses all the elements that go into your stand against cancer.

In choosing your composition, you must be particularly thoughtful taking into consideration the feelings of your loved ones as well as the guidance of your medical team. The choices you make not only affect you but also the people around you. What you need to understand is that you can choose to be optimistic and positive in your presentation to the world regardless of your disease status or situation. And of course, no matter what "song" you chose yesterday, today is a new day. As the headlining act in your own show, you have the right to modify your song selection anytime you like.

> You can choose to be optimistic in your stand against cancer!

Choosing Your Arrangement

A song may have many different arrangements (or versions) that have been written by composers and/or performers to reflect their personal interpretation of the original piece. For example, a composer or performer might choose to extend the song by adding an extra solo, verse, or chorus. Or, he or she might decide to write a version of the song that can be played on a different instrument than was originally intended. The result of modifications such as these is a new arrangement of the song.

Once a song has been selected, the musician needs to decide on the arrangement that best suits his or her personality. In life, your "arrangement" is your own personal touch to your song, and more specifically it is a way of holding on to your personality and your sense of self during your stand against cancer. While many people with cancer thus may share the same song or outlook on life (i.e., an optimistic attitude), your arrangement is specific to you. It is how you choose to express and channel your personality through your disposition. For example, if you have an optimistic outlook on your life with cancer and have an outgoing and gregarious personality, your arrangement might lead you down the path of cancer advocacy, lobbying for changes in government health policies. On the other hand, if you have an optimistic outlook on life and have a more introverted personality, your arrangement might lead you down the path of volunteering one-on-one with patients, or participating in small cancer support groups. While any "song" and "arrangement" you choose to present to the world is valid in your journey with cancer, staying true to yourself and your personality throughout this process is key. The bottom line—don't let cancer disrupt your sense of self.

> Regardless of your disease status, let your personality shine through!

Choosing the Details of Your Performance

Once a musician has selected a song and an arrangement, it's on to the performance! Your life performance is your chance to show the world who you are and what you stand for. The details of your performance, including the location (your preferred surroundings), the venue that best suits your personality (your preferred lifestyle), and the audience you wish to reach (your family, friends, and others), are all important considerations that impact your quality of life with cancer. Just as a musician will take certain steps to ensure a smooth and flawless show, you can set the stage for having a good quality of life with cancer by being relaxed in your surroundings, maintaining a comfortable lifestyle, and keeping good company with family and friends. A good quality of life will help you live life to the fullest, regardless of your disease status.

Your Life Performance and the Meaning of Cancer

Music and the performing arts can help you understand the meaning of cancer in your life. As alluded to in Chapter 15, some of the most effective pieces of music and/or theatrical art have the power to elicit emotions and feelings on a level far beyond the ordinary. This is not to say that these art forms hold the secret to life, however, they are able to show you the complex patterns of connectivity that exist in the world, and by doing so can provide you with reasonable explanations to some of life's most difficult questions. In other words, these works of art are able to show you the bigger picture in life at a time when your mind might not otherwise make sense of things on its own. Although it is rare to make connections with powerful art forms, when it happens it can literally change your outlook on life.

In searching for the meaning of life, or more precisely the meaning of life with cancer, my patients often ask me that very difficult question, "Why me? Why do I have cancer?" Early in my career, I misinterpreted this query as a form of denial, but over the years I have come to realize that this is a perfectly valid question. Although sometimes there is an obvious answer (i.e., the case of a long-term smoker developing lung cancer), the majority of the time an obvious answer simply does not exist. For years I looked (and listened) for a meaningful response to this delicate question, but despite the deepest of soul searching I made little if any progress on this front. However, recently I have found a clue hidden deep in music that has lead me closer to the truth, and through this connection I have experienced one of those rare life-changing epiphanies that I would like to share with you here.

> The truth is that life is not always fair, but good things can come out of even the worst of circumstances. For example, there is nothing fair about a teenager passing away from leukemia at the age of 19, but, as we learned in Chapter 4, even tragic endings like this one can lead to wonderful beginnings and incredible stories of hope and inspiration (i.e., the formation of the T.J. Martell Foundation). How does cancer lead to great things? Cancer brings out the best in people and brings communities together. Like a thread intricately woven within the fabric of life, this 19-year-old teenager touched the lives of all of those around him. His disease affected not only himself but was also felt by society as a whole. And from powerful connections like this one, people unite and great things are created.

Personally, my life-changing connection (my epiphany) with music came one day when I was listening to the lyrics from the Rush song, "Limelight" written by Neil Peart. Although I had listened to this song many times in my life, it was at that moment that I first grasped the powerful nature of his lyrics and the deep meaning behind this song. In the last verse, Peart concludes that, "All the world's indeed a stage" and all of us are simply "each another's audience." Looking at life in this light, each of us is our own playwright and a performer on the stage of life, and every day our story is being written in the people we meet, the places we visit, and the memories we create. What is truly incredible about these lyrics is that in an indescribable way, they put life into perspective—as if to show us that the difficulties we face every day are just another scene in our play, and that "they too will come to pass."

Peart's powerful lyrical concept in "Limelight" is a direct modern day adaptation from Jaques' soliloquy in William Shakespeare's play, "As You Like It." This play emerged in the late 1500s or early 1600s, and boasts one of the most famous theatrical monologues of all time. Act II, Scene 7, reads:

> All the world's a stage,
> And all the men and women merely players:
> They have their exits and their entrances;
> And one man in his time plays many parts,
> His acts being seven ages. At first the infant,
> Mewling and puking in the nurse's arms.
> And then the whining school-boy, with his satchel
> And shining morning face, creeping like snail
> Unwillingly to school. And then the lover,
> Sighing like furnace, with a woeful ballad
> Made to his mistress' eyebrow. Then a soldier,
> Full of strange oaths and bearded like the pard,
> Jealous in honour, sudden and quick in quarrel,
> Seeking the bubble reputation
> Even in the cannon's mouth. And then the justice,
> In fair round belly with good capon lined,

With eyes severe and beard of formal cut,
Full of wise saws and modern instances;
And so he plays his part. The sixth age shifts
Into the lean and slipper'd pantaloon,
With spectacles on nose and pouch on side,
His youthful hose, well saved, a world too wide
For his shrunk shank; and his big manly voice,
Turning again toward childish treble, pipes
And whistles in his sound. Last scene of all,
That ends this strange eventful history,
Is second childishness and mere oblivion,
Sans teeth, sans eyes, sans taste, sans everything.

There are many interpretations behind the meaning of Jaques' soliloquy, however, most agree that the "seven ages" binds together the fragments that make up life, and by doing so show us the many truths of existence. Shakespeare eloquently puts into words the concept that from childhood until old age, we have roles that we naturally play out in life. He describes these roles in an almost matter-of-fact fashion, and his use of chronological order provides a sense of continuity to the listener. Yet, his commentary on life reaches far deeper than simply outlining the aging process.

In addition to defining the roles we play out in life, the "seven ages" monologue provides us with explanations of some of the most difficult questions we face on a daily basis. As if looking through a crystal ball, this soliloquy reassures the listener that where you are in life is exactly where you should be, and that the seemingly isolated events of the world are part of a more complex and interconnected story. The beauty of theater in this regard is that it is able to address challenging topics in a tender way that is soothing for the soul. Instead of providing a direct answer to the question, "Why do I have cancer?" Shakespeare seems to gently encourage a sense of acceptance and understanding of the situation. And in a subtle fashion, he shows us the bigger picture of life and how our life performances are all connected in this world. After all, in the words of Shakespeare, "All the world's a stage."

It's a delicate thing to say, but your diagnosis affects all of us, and it means something to the world. Let music and art help you find meaning behind your diagnosis of cancer.

By incorporating music and art in your life, you will become more connected to your partner, family, friends, loved ones, caregivers, and community, and you will be more aware of the important role you play in the bigger picture of life. While this may not directly answer the question of why you have cancer, hopefully it will provide you with an understanding of the deeper meaning behind your cancer.

You possess the skills and abilities necessary to stand up to your cancer, and music and art can help you in your journey. Although cancer has made an appearance in your life performance, you are the star of your show and have the power to script the future 'as you like it.' Use this opportunity to minimize the role cancer will play in your production, and live life to the fullest while finding the balance between art and science in your life. And although mistakes will happen along the way, make them loud and make them count, and drop them and move on. Because no matter what, your song keeps playing, and time keeps passing. Just as musicians spend a significant amount of time practicing their parts prior to each performance, each day is a learning process and an opportunity to make a difference in your life and in the life of others. Focus on maintaining a good quality of life as you move forward in your journey, and remember that your audience is all around you, every day in everything you do, and everywhere you go. Cancer or not, we are all in this together.

CHAPTER 17

Finale

Nimesh P. Nagarsheth, MD

On behalf of the N.E.D. project, my fellow bandmates and I would like to thank you for taking the time to listen to our thoughts and ideas about the incredible healing powers of music as it relates to cancer. We truly hope our words and stories of inspiration have been able to touch you in a meaningful way, and we sincerely wish you the best as you move forward in your journey of life.

As the story goes, N.E.D. began in a small hotel conference room in Tampa, Florida in March 2008 with a couple of acoustic guitars, a pair of drumsticks on a padded chair, untrained voices, and a dream of using the power of music to help heal cancer. Breaking tradition and starting with just a handful of supporters, N.E.D. forged ahead and never looked back. In terms of miracles, we are still in disbelief that as six busy surgeons scattered across the United States, we were somehow able to convince a record company (and publisher for that matter) to invest in this unprecedented (and quite frankly, risky) idea. However, throughout our ups and downs, we never lost hope, and thanks to the incredible support of people just like you, we have seen our dream become a reality. With the release of our album and this book just over 1 year later, the N.E.D. project is now officially up and running and fully functional.

So where do we go from here? Our vision for the possibilities of N.E.D. takes us far beyond improving cancer awareness, education, quality of life, and fundraising through the mediums of music and literature. We view N.E.D. as the start of a new movement—an in-depth and ongoing project that will lead to significant contributions and improvements in the areas of cancer prevention, screening, early detection, diagnosis and treatment, as well as research. We invite you to join us as we build this N.E.D. movement in the fight against cancer. Reaching the community in novel ways and breaking the mold when it comes to the traditional barriers of medicine is just the beginning. Now more than ever, with your help, anything is possible. Together we have the power to shape the future and define a new approach to cancer care in the 21st century.

For ourselves and for our patients, N.E.D. has become more than just a disease state or the name of a band; N.E.D. has become a way of life. These inspiring words (or initials) are music to the ears of all those who wish to listen, and they reach deep within the mind, body, and soul. Possessing tremendous strength in terms of uniting people behind a cause and motivating people to maintain a healthy quality of life, N.E.D., just like music, sends a universal message of hope to patients, loved ones, and caregivers.

In the near future, look for the creation of the N.E.D. Cancer Foundation that will be dedicated to the complete care of the gynecologic cancer patient. Holding true to our roots, this foundation will harness the energy and power from various forms of media to help us fulfill our goals and the mission of the ever-expanding N.E.D. project. Stay tuned for the next phase in our exciting journey, and in the meantime remember that the secret to successfully moving forward in your life with cancer may be closer than you think.

Listen to more music . . .

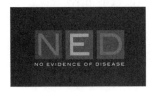

Encore: A Message from the President of Motéma Music

Listening to music deeply, and letting the body and mind follow the flow of the beat, can help you unlock your emotional vault. Although tears may flow, anger may bubble up, or passions may rise, the release of that honest emotion can be just what the doctor ordered.

Deep listening in and of itself is a healing activity. Check it out for yourself. Try listening closely to a room you are in. Listen for the sounds and listen for the silence behind the sounds. Listen to the rhythmic and melodic relationships between everything you hear. Whether you are at a symphony hall, listening to music in your living room, or in a hospital bed listening to the beep and huff of a respirator, you will find that every sound has a relationship to every other sound, and also to the silence underlying the sound. Consciously tuning into these subtle sound relationships can be incredibly soothing for the soul. Through deep listening, I have discovered that even "difficult" sounds such as sirens or jackhammers have a peaceful place in life's symphony, and thus no longer cause me stress.

Although I have been lucky enough not to develop cancer, if I ever did, the first thing I would do is go to a specialist and seek the help and advice from experts in the field. At the same time, I would look within, and immerse myself in music that felt healing to me. I would swim in those rhythms every day, doing my best to heal myself from the inside out with music, while my doctors worked on healing me from the outside in with their skills and tools.

If you are suffering from cancer, I want to help you heal from the inside out. Please connect with me through the contact information below, and I will personally send you some music to help you on your healing journey. Motéma musicians truly care about making heart connections through music, and are hand-picked for the label. I would be honored to be a part of your healing process.

Sincerely,
Jana Herzen
President
Motéma Music
New York, NY
www.motema.com

Glossary of Medical Terms

Attending physician: A doctor who has completed his or her medical training in a specific specialty and actively practices medicine in that specialty.

Brachytherapy: A type of radiation treatment where the radioactive source is placed inside or very close to the tissue being treated.

Cancer: A disease in which cells grow uncontrollably, invade into surrounding tissues or organs, and have the potential to metastasize (spread).

Chemobrain: The cognitive impairment that occurs in some patients that has been associated with chemotherapy and possibly cancer itself.

Chemotherapy: Drugs designed to kill cancer cells, to keep them from growing, or to keep them from multiplying.

Clinical trial (also clinical study): A research study that investigates the value and effectiveness of new medical approaches. For cancer-related research, this typically involves a new screening, prevention, diagnosis, or treatment strategy.

Debulking: The surgical removal of a malignant tumor.

Electrocardiogram (also ECG or EKG): The graphical depiction of the electrical activity of the heart.

Fellow: A doctor that has completed training in at least one area of specialization and is in training for an additional sub-specialized area.

Intern: A physician in training who is in his or her first year of residency.

Laparoscopic surgery (also minimally invasive surgery): A surgical technique that uses video and/or digital technology to perform surgery through small incisions as compared the larger incisions utilized in traditional "open" surgery. Patients undergoing laparoscopic surgery benefit from less perioperative pain and an overall quicker recovery period.

M & M (also Morbidity and Mortality Conference): A departmental medical conference held at regular intervals at most major medical centers in which doctors freely discuss and review medical complications and medical errors.

Radiation therapy: Medical use of radiation to control and destroy cancer cells.

Resident: A doctor in training for an area of specialization after completing medical school.

Robotic surgery: The use of robots to assist with surgery.

Scientific method: An organized set of techniques designed to investigate a phenomena which includes formulating and testing a hypothesis.

Targeted therapy: Drugs and other substances that are designed to block the growth or kill cancer cells by targeting specific molecules within these cells.

Tumor: An abnormal swelling or growth.

Glossary of Musical Terms

A theme: The original musical idea.

B theme: The secondary musical idea.

Bach: Usually refers to Johann Sebastian, 1685–1750, a member of an outstanding family of musicians.

Bar: A unit of measurement in music.

Baroque: Period in music history (1600–1750) known for its decorative ornamentation.

Beat: Pulse or count.

Bebop: A period in American Jazz roughly early-1940s to mid-1950s.

Beethoven: An unusual musical mind, 1770–1827, Germany and perhaps the world's most famous composer.

Big band: An American phenomena (early-1930s to late-1940s); making a comeback; Duke Ellington was the premier big band leader.

Bridge: A transition idea usually leading (a connector) from one theme to another.

C theme: A third theme or musical idea; usually in connection with the rondo form.

Chord: Two or more notes sounding together.

Classical music: Basically, music that is written down and played the same way each time. Broadly includes music from the 9th century to present times.

Common time: Music in 4/4 time; music with four beats and the quarter notes equals one of the four beats. It is the most used time signature for modern popular music.

Dixieland: A style of popular American music; manifestations of early jazz associated with the city of New Orleans.

Dizzy Gillespie: Jazz trumpet player, bandleader, and innovator in the bebop movement.

Gig: A musical job.

Groove: A neat musical idea that fits together and can be interchanged with other ideas. A feeling of the beat.

Handel: George Frederick, 1685–1759, contemporary of J.S. Bach.

Harmony: Two or more sounds or processes together.

Haydn: Franz Josef, 1709–1832; one of the great idea persons in music who influenced Beethoven and Mozart.

Heavy metal music: Phenomena of the 20th century; grew out of the "rock" movement; "raucous rock".

Improvisation: Music created "on the spot;" instant ideas similar to speaking on a subject without preparation notes; primarily based on creating ideas from a first idea; it is not fixed on a page, but flexible; the core element that is jazz.

Intro: Short for introduction but commonly used in music to refer to the opening idea.

Jazz: Has at its core "improvisation." As a musical phenomenon, jazz centers on freedom of expression; the ideas can be freely stated, enhanced, or changed. Change is the heart of jazz whereas meticulous recreation is the heart of classical style; both use the same notes.

Marimba: Wooden bars played over resonators which originated as the African straw fiddle.

Measure: Sometimes called a bar in music. It is also the fundamental process involved in music performance.

Melody: An idea in sound.

Metronome: A mechanical device to aid in the measuring process.

Note: A characteristic musical sound. There are seven of them in western music.

Outro (also outtro): Two things; the opposite of intro and what happens at the conclusion of a selection.

Percussion: Music created by slow to rapid reiteration. An object that makes a sound when struck, shaken, stirred, or by any other method that causes it to vibrate.

Piano: Dynamic meaning quiet or a keyboard instrument: i.e., the piano.

Pythagoras: One of the most famous ancient Greek philosophers considered the Father of Music Therapy.

Rest: Measured silence.

Rock music: Outgrowth from spiritual blues and rhythm and blues.

Rhythm (meter/tempo): The movement of anything. Meter which means "to measure," establishes or defines dimension. Meter is the measurement of anything. Tempo is the speed of anything.

Sight reading: Playing only and exactly what you see, typically on the spot without any preparation.

Solo: A single voice.

Sound: An audible vibration that is transmitted through mediums such as a liquid, solid, or gas.

Swing: Outgrowth from the period in American music referred to as Big Band Jazz; an alteration of rhythm from strict and stately to casual.

Woodblock: A drum made out of wood; a slit drum.

APPENDIX IV

Cancer Resources and Contact Information

Oral Cavity and Pharynx
The Roswell Park Cancer Institute
Elm & Carlton Streets
Buffalo, NY 14263
877.275.7724
www.roswellpark.org/Patient_Care/Types_of_Cancer/Head_NeckCenter

Digestive System
American College of Gastroenterology
PO Box 342260
Bethesda, MD 20827-2260
301.263.9000
www.acg.go.org

GIST Support International
12 Bomaca Drive
Doylestown, PA 18901
215.340.9374
www.gistsupport.org

Respiratory System
The Bonnie J. Addario Lung Cancer Foundation
San Francisco, CA
415.357.1278
www.thelungcancerfoundation.org

Lung Cancer Online
www.lungcanceronline.org

Skin
The Skin Cancer Foundation
149 Madison Avenue
Suite 901
New York, NY 10016
212.725.5176
www.skincancer.org

American Melanoma Foundation
4150 Regents Park Row
Suite 300
La Jolla, CA 92037
858.882.7712
www.melanomafoundation.org

Breast
Share: Self-help for Women with Breast or Ovarian Cancer
1501 Broadway
Suite 704A
New York, NY 10036
866.891.2392
www.sharecancersupport.org

Susan G. Koman for the Cure
5005 LBJ Freeway
Suite 250
Dallas, TX 75244
877.465.6636
www.komen.org

Genital (Female)
Cancer Schmancer Movement
New York, NY
www.cancerschmancer.org

Gynecologic Cancer Foundation
230 W. Monroe
Suite 2528
Chicago, IL 60606
800.444.4441
www.thegcf.org

N.E.D. Cancer Foundation
New York, NY
www.nedcancerfoundation.org

The Ovarian Cancer Research Fund
14 Pennsylvania Plaza
Suite 1400
New York, NY 10122
212.268.1002
www.ocrf.org

Genital (Male)
American Prostate Society
1340-F Charwood Road
Hanover, MD 21076
410.859.3735
www.ameripros.org

American Urological Association Foundation
Patient Education
1000 Corporate Blvd.
Linthicum, MD 21090
410.689.3700
www.auafoundation.org

Urinary System
Kidney Cancer Association
PO Box 96503
Washington, DC 20090
800.850.9132
kidney.cancer@hotmail.com
www.kidneycancerassociation.org

Bladder Cancer Advocacy Network
4813 St. Elmo Avenue
Bethesda, MD 20814
301.215.9099 or 888.901.2226
www.bcan.org

Brain and Nervous System
American Brain Tumor Association
2720 River Road
Des Plaines, IL 60018
847.827.9910 or 800.886.2282
Fax: 847.827.9918
info@abta.org
www.abta.org

National Brain Tumor Society
East Cost Office:
124 Watertown Street
Suite 2D
Watertown, MA 02472
617.924.9997
Fax: 617.924.9998
West Coast Office:
22 Battery Street
Suite 612
San Francisco, CA 94111-5524
415.834.9970
Fax: 415.834.9980
info@braintumor.org
www.braintumor.org

Endocrine
The Ohio State University Comprehensive Cancer Center
James Cancer Hospital and Solove Research Institute
300 W. 10th Avenue
Columbus, OH 43210
800.293.5066
www.jamesline.com/cancertypes/endocrine/about/Pages/index.aspx

Lymphoma
Lymphoma Research Foundation
East Coast Office:
115 Broadway
13th Floor
New York, New York 10006
212.349.2910
Fax: 212.349.2886
West Coast Office:
8800 Venice Blvd.
Suite 207
Los Angeles, CA 90034
310.204.7040
Fax: 310.204.7043
helpline@lymphoma.org
www.lymphoma.org

The Leukemia & Lymphoma Society
800.955.4572
www.leukemia-lymphoma.org

Leukemia
Leukemia Research Foundation
3520 Lake Avenue
Suite 202
Wilmette, IL 60091
847.424.0600
Fax: 847.424.0606
www.leukemia-research.org

Others
American Cancer Society
800.227.2345
www.cancer.org

CancerCare
275 Seventh Avenue
New York, New York 10001
800.813.4673
Fax: 212.712.8495
info@cancercare.org
www.cancercare.org

Gilda's Club Worldwide
48 Wall Street
11th Floor
New York, New York 10005
888.GILDA.4U
Fax: 917.305.0549
info@gildasclub.org
www.gildasclub.org

National Cancer Institute
NCI Public Inquiries Office
6116 Executive Blvd.
Room 3036A
Bethesda, MD 20892-8322
800.422.6237
cancergovstaff@mail.nih.gov
www.cancer.gov

National Coalition for Cancer Survivorship
1010 Wayne Avenue
Suite 770
Silver Spring, MD 20910
301.650.9127 or 888.650.9127
Fax: 301.565.9670
info@canceradvocacy.org
www.canceradvocacy.org

The Wellness Community
919 18th Street
NW Suite 54
Washington, DC 20006
202.659.9709 or 888.793.9355
Fax: 202.659.9301
help@thewellnesscommunity.org
www.thewellnesscommunity.org

Index

participation in organizations, 146
resources for, 143–145, 148
volunteering as, 146
isolation, emotional, 103, 105, 121

J

Jacobs model, of grief, 41, 43
jazz, American
forms of, 4, 6, 30, 158
healthcare funding and, 32–38
history of, 29–30
Jazz Foundation of America, 32–33, 35
jazz improvisation, 93–94, 134
medicine and, 29–38
"Jazz Therapy" (Motema Music), 34–35
Joel, Billy, 141–143
journaling, of grief process, 44

K

knowledge, power of, 54–55, 105
Kubler-Ross model, of grief, 41–42, 43, 47

L

Laennec, Rene, 14, 16
laparoscopic surgery, 114, 132
Latimer, Jim, 4, 12–13, 53, 81
leap second, 161
learning
artistic approaches to, 54–55, 139
from mistakes, 92, 95–98, 196
music as medium for, 24–25, 66, 70–71
leave of absence, from work, 127, 128
legal counsel/issues
for end-of-life planning, 168, 169–171
partner's role in, 124, 126–128
life balance
inner, music as tool for, 87–90
timing in, 151, 157, 160–161
life with cancer. See also quality of life
finding meaning of, 189–190, 192–196
prepare for unexpected in, 168, 181–187
time estimates for, 155–156

lifestyle
benefits of maintaining, 56–57, 59–60, 151, 192
partner's role in, 109, 112
"Limelight" (Peart), 194
listening
art of, 24, 71, 102
coping power of, 72–73, 90
creating music vs., 22–23, 38, 89
as partner's role, 109, 112, 117
live performance, 189–196
arrangement for, 189, 191–192
composition for, 189, 190–191
details for, 189, 192
meaning of cancer and, 189–190, 192–196
mistakes during, 92–95, 160
opportunities provided by, 102, 189
preparation rituals for, 189–190
unexpected challenges with, 179–181
living will, 126, 168, 170–171
loss. See grief/grieving

M

mammogram, 147
Martell, Tony, 35–37
mathematics, music derived from, 10, 11, 19
meaning of life, with cancer, 189–190, 192–196
measure, in music, 101–102, 157
measuring, in music process, 12
medical appointments, 109, 112
medical bills, non-covered, 108, 119, 125–126
medical conditions, acute care for, 173–174
medical history, keeping notebook of, 73
medical schools, humanistic programs of, 49, 84, 87, 88
medical team
for cancer treatment, 31, 80, 106–107, 116, 118
personal choices affecting, 104, 190–191
Medicare/Medicaid, 125